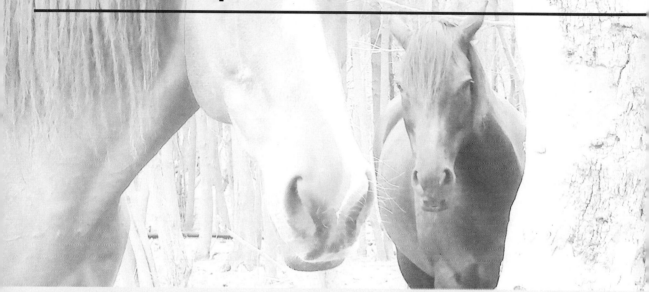

Fascial Anatomy
of the Equine Forelimb

Fascial Anatomy of the Equine Forelimb

CARLA M. LUSI AND HELEN M. S. DAVIES

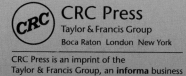

CRC Press
Taylor & Francis Group
Boca Raton London New York

CRC Press is an imprint of the
Taylor & Francis Group, an **informa** business

CRC Press
Taylor & Francis Group
6000 Broken Sound Parkway NW, Suite 300
Boca Raton, FL 33487-2742

© 2018 by Taylor & Francis Group, LLC
CRC Press is an imprint of Taylor & Francis Group, an Informa business

No claim to original U.S. Government works

Printed on acid-free paper

Printed and bound in India by Replika Press Pvt. Ltd.

International Standard Book Number-13: 978-0-8153-8744-2 (Hardback)
International Standard Book Number-13: 978-0-8153-8738-1 (Paperback)

Visit the Taylor & Francis Web site at
http://www.taylorandfrancis.com

and the CRC Press Web site at
http://www.crcpress.com

CONTENTS

Preface   ix
Authors   xi

CHAPTER 1   **UNDERSTANDING THE FASCIAL SYSTEM**   1

INTRODUCTION   1
WHAT IS FASCIA?   1
    Composition and structure   1
    Identifying fascia   2
PAST INVESTIGATIONS OF THE EQUINE FASCIAL SYSTEM   3
REFERENCES   3
BIBLIOGRAPHY   4

CHAPTER 2   **ANATOMY OF THE EQUINE FORELIMB**   5

THE PROXIMAL FORELIMB   5
THE DISTAL FORELIMB   11
PASSIVE SUPPORT OF THE FORELIMB   13
LIGAMENTS AND SOFT TISSUES OF THE DISTAL FORELIMB   14
    Joint capsules   14
    Sesamoidean ligaments   14
    Flexor tendons   14
    Extensor tendons   16
    Annular ligaments   17
REFERENCES   17
BIBLIOGRAPHY   17

CHAPTER 3   **FASCIA OF THE EQUINE METACARPUS AND PROXIMAL PORTION OF THE DIGIT**   19

INTRODUCTION   19
SUPERFICIAL FASCIA   20
    General findings   20
    Dorsal, medial and lateral aspects   21
    Palmar aspect   28

DEEP FASCIA   32
   Dorsal, medial and lateral aspects   32
   Palmar aspect   41
FASCIA OF THE CARPAL FLEXOR TENDON SHEATH   42
REFERENCES   46
BIBLIOGRAPHY   46

CHAPTER 4   **FASCIA OF THE EQUINE ANTEBRACHIUM**   **49**

INTRODUCTION   49
ANTEBRACHIAL FASCIA: SUMMARY   50
SUPERFICIAL FASCIA   53
   Medial aspect   53
   Caudal and lateral aspects   58
DEEP FASCIA   65
   Cranial compartment   65
   Craniolateral compartment   70
   Lateral compartment   73
   Caudal compartments   76
   Carpal retinacula and tendon sheaths   87
REFERENCES   91
BIBLIOGRAPHY   92

CHAPTER 5   **FASCIA OF THE EQUINE SHOULDER GIRDLE AND BRACHIUM**   **93**

INTRODUCTION   93
SUPERFICIAL FASCIA   94
   General findings   94
   Continuity and attachment   94
DEEP FASCIA   103
   General findings   103
LATERAL ASPECT   103
   Superficial lamina   103
   Deep lamina   110
MEDIAL ASPECT   121
   Superficial lamina   121
   Deep lamina   123
REFERENCES   137
BIBLIOGRAPHY   137

CHAPTER 6	**FASCIAL LINES EXTENDING INTO THE HOOF**	**139**
	INTRODUCTION	139
	SUPERFICIAL FASCIA	140
	DEEP FASCIA	144
	CONCLUSION	152
	REFERENCES	154
CHAPTER 7	**FASCIAL LINES OF TENSION IN THE EQUINE FORELIMB**	**155**
	INTRODUCTION	155
	SUMMARY	156
	Flexion/extension of the digit	156
	Flexion/extension of the fetlock joint	158
	Flexion/extension of the carpus, elbow and shoulder	161
	Fascial force transmission in adult horse limbs	162
	UNDERSTANDING PASSIVE MOVEMENT COORDINATION	162
	REFERENCES	164
	BIBLIOGRAPHY	165
Index		**167**

Over the past decade, there has been an increased interest in the fascial system of the human body and how it contributes to movement and injury progression. In endeavouring to understand and improve locomotory abnormalities and dysfunction, many human practitioners have adopted a more holistic approach in which lines of fascial connectivity and integration are visualised and targeted during treatment.

The recent identification of fascial lines in humans has provided a visual map which helps practitioners to see the relatedness of structures and track the development of compensatory postural adjustments or pain that result from dysfunction in otherwise unsuspected areas of the body. Hence, it brings attention to the fact that improper loading of particular structures, or an inability of a structure to effectively manage loads, may be related to a restriction or locomotor abnormality somewhere else in the body.

Past equine anatomical works have focused largely on the musculoskeletal system and have overlooked the anatomy and connecting role of the fascia. Hence, there is limited literature available directed at the equine fascial system and its role in contributing to, or enhancing, musculoskeletal function.

The purpose of this book is therefore to provide a visual atlas of the fascial connectivity in the equine forelimb – an area that is commonly fraught with injury in both pleasure and performance horses. In doing so, this work aims to provide both the clinician and the horse owner with a detailed anatomical reference that aids in the understanding and management of forelimb locomotor problems. In addition, paths of forelimb fascial continuity identified in this book provide a foundation for further studies of fascial continuity beyond the forelimb.

Images provided in this book have been prepared using gross dissection techniques performed on fresh equine forelimbs. These images are each accompanied by reference images to help readers orientate themselves with different aspects of the equine forelimb. The basic musculoskeletal anatomy of the forelimb described in the first chapter will further assist readers with developing a complete picture of the forelimb functional anatomy.

The functional significance of fascial characteristics highlighted in this book is discussed throughout each chapter and is based on both the available research completed on the fascial and musculoskeletal systems in humans, and the general principles of biomechanics. Our aim is that these short discussions will encourage readers to think of load distribution and postural stability in the forelimb as things that are dependent on the connectivity enabled by the fascial system, rather than on individual bones, muscles or joints. Thus, we hope this book leads horse owners and practitioners to a broader understanding of equine forelimb biomechanics and locomotor abnormalities.

Carla M. Lusi and Helen M. S. Davies

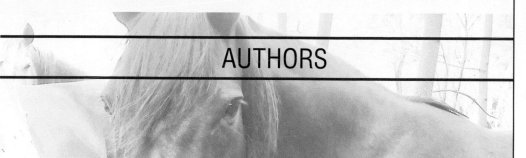

AUTHORS

Carla M. Lusi (BSc, PhD) completed a Bachelor of Science at the University of Melbourne. Her PhD (supervised by Helen M. S. Davies) focused on mapping out the fascial connectivity in the equine forelimb.

Helen M. S. Davies (BAgSci. MAgrSc. BVSc. PhD) is Associate Professor in Veterinary Anatomy at the University of Melbourne. She was previously the primary author on three anatomy chapters in *Equine Podiatry* (publ. Saunders 2007) and coauthored a chapter on hoof biomechanics in *Equine Laminitis* (publ. Wiley 2016). She has extensive experience in teaching veterinary locomotory and regional anatomy to veterinary students and post graduate courses in physiotherapy and other associated professions (25 years); equine biomechanical and anatomical research (25 years); training horses and riders in all disciplines (40 years); treating and advising trainers and riders on the prevention and management of musculoskeletal conditions (25 years); and measuring the development of changes in forelimb loading in young horses in training (25 years).

CHAPTER 1

UNDERSTANDING THE FASCIAL SYSTEM

INTRODUCTION

In trying to determine ways in which load distribution and postural stability of the fetlock joint is managed, the recent interest around the function and importance of fascia is of particular relevance. Although it is considered to have several mechanical and physiological roles, the clinical importance of the fascia as a system comes down to how it integrates all systems of the body and how this understanding can be used to direct treatment, rehabilitation, and exercise in order to prevent injury or catastrophic breakdown of an individual musculoskeletal element.

The identification of fascial lines in humans has not provided solutions to all musculoskeletal injuries; however, it has provided a visual map which has helped practitioners to see the relatedness of structures and the development of compensatory postural adjustments or pain that result from dysfunction in otherwise unsuspected areas of the body. Hence, it brings attention to the fact that improper loading of the joint, or an inability of the joint to effectively manage loads, may be related to a restriction or locomotor abnormality somewhere else in the body.

In horses, investigation of the body-wide fascial connections and meridians is a large undertaking as there is a very limited amount of literature available that is directed at the equine fascial system (described further in the following). However, identifying paths of fascial continuity in individual body segments (such as the forelimb) may provide a foundation upon which further studies looking at fascial continuity can be based.

WHAT IS FASCIA?

Composition and structure

The fascial system refers to a body-wide connective tissue matrix, which provides structural support to all bodily tissues and organs, as well as communicating pathways within and between these structures. In investigating the structure and composition of fascia, there are three components to be considered. These include its cellular anatomy, the fibres it comprises, and its extracellular matrix.

The cellular component of fascia consists of fibroblasts, adipocytes, macrophages, mast cells, undifferentiated mesenchymal cells, plasma cells and leukocytes. The most abundant of these cells are the fibroblasts, which are under endocrine control and are responsible for the synthesis of complex carbohydrates, collagen and elastic fibres, as well as other proteins of the extracellular matrix.

It has been shown that strain and pressure applied to fascia stimulates the proliferation of fibroblasts and causes them to orientate along the same stress lines as the direction of applied force (Gehlsen, Ganion, & Helfst, 1991). This process is mediated by changes in the internal cytoskeletal structure, which similarly respond to the tensional forces applied to them. Hence, it is implied that mechanical stresses placed on the body influence the overall composition and structure of the fascia, causing it to adapt via an increased production of fibroblasts and rearrangement of the internal cytoskeletal structure.

The fibrillar component of fascia includes two main fibre types: collagen and elastin. Generally, collagen fibres are flexible in an unloaded state but become stiff and strong when subject to tension. This tension and resulting strength is provided by covalent cross links between collagen molecules, which develop and arrange according to the direction and magnitude of mechanical loads applied to them (Hukins & Aspden, 1985; Stecco, 2015). The alignment of the collagen fibre itself is usually along lines of tensile stress and hence can be indicative of loading patterns and function.

In contrast, elastic fibres are comprised of two different structural components including elastin and microfibrils. Elastic fibres differ in function to collagen fibres in that they provide tissues with the required resilience to transient stretch. They have the ability to be stretched up to 150% of their original length in response to applied force and recoil to their original length when force is removed. Long collagen fibres, which can only stretch <10% of their resting length prior to tearing, are usually interwoven with elastic fibres to prevent overstretching and rupture.

The last component of the fascial system is the extracellular matrix. This functions to distribute mechanical stresses and provide a structural framework for the adherence and movement of cells and comprises both elastic and collagen fibres, as well as ground substance. The ground substance refers to an amorphous gel-like substance surrounding the cellular and fibrillar components of fascia and which functions to provide support and nutrition to all cells. Its water content, and thus viscosity, determines the overall mobility and connectivity of the connective tissue matrix and allows for movement of adjacent fibres with limited friction. Proteoglycans, hyaluronic acid and link proteins are the primary constituents of the ground substance.

Identifying fascia

The organisation of fascia, its expansive connectivity and its varying physical characteristics (thickness, composition etc.) introduces a lot of area for debate and confusion when it comes to distinguishing and describing its anatomy and function. Generally, it is accepted that the fascia of the human body can be categorised into the fascia superficialis (superficial fascia) and the fascia profunda (deep fascia). This nomenclature remains consistent in regards to the equine fascial system.

Both types of fascia are made up of the same constituents described earlier; however, their relative proportions differ greatly. The superficial fascia exists as a layer of loose areolar connective tissue situated beneath the dermis of the skin, which varies in thickness and composition along different locations depending on its functional role. Fibrous septa, which connect the superficial fascia to both the overlying skin and the underlying deep fascia, allows the superficial fascia a role in maintaining the integrity of the skin and in supporting subcutaneous structures.

The superficial fascia is comprised of interwoven collagen fibres, loosely packed and mixed with an abundance of elastic fibres. These elastic fibres allow for displacement between the superficial fascia layer and neighbouring tissue layers, thereby allowing sliding between tissue planes with movement and muscular activity. In some regions, the superficial fascia further acts as a subdividing tissue plane, which forms compartments around major subcutaneous vessels.

In contrast the deep fascia refers to fibrous fascial sheets, which not only envelop and separate muscles, but also forms sheaths around vessels and nerves and provides a means of strengthening ligaments around joints. Essentially, the deep fascia binds all structures together.

Two types of deep fascia have been described including the aponeurotic deep fascia and the epimysial deep fascia. The aponeurotic fascia refers to all the 'well-defined fibrous sheaths that cover and keep in place a group of muscles or serve for the insertion of a broad muscle.' It remains separated from underlying muscles and is capable of transmitting forces over a long distance due to its thickness (590–1453 μm) and well-defined fibre orientation. According to its position and function, it may adhere to, or become continuous with, the periosteum of bones, the paratenon of tendons and ligaments, or the connective tissue comprising joint capsules. Such examples in humans include the thoracolumbar fascia and the investing fascia compartmentalising the muscles of the limbs.

The epimysial fascia refers to the thinner, yet still well organised, deep fascia, which is strongly connected to muscles and allows them to slide against overlying tissue planes. In contrast to the aponeurotic fascia, it is specific to each muscle, providing a medium for insertion of muscle fibres and giving off fibrous septa that penetrate the muscle. Hence, it transmits forces generated by single muscle fibres and has a more localised range of action.

PAST INVESTIGATIONS OF THE EQUINE FASCIAL SYSTEM

There has been very little research published concerning the functional anatomy of the equine fascial system and how it may be targeted to improve and optimise movement and performance. In fact most veterinary anatomy textbooks present the musculoskeletal system as one that is comprised of anatomically and functionally distinct units (either skeletal or muscular), often completely ignoring the integrative role of fascia. As a result, information on the equine fascial system is inconsistent, incomplete or difficult to access (see reference list at end of chapter).

The benefits of recognising the fascial system in human movement and performance suggests that the equine fascial system provides an area for research with lots of potential for improving equine performance and managing and preventing injury. The main aim of this book is to encourage thinking about related movements (which are enabled via the fascial system) and how movement restrictions or abnormalities in one area of the body may result in load redistribution and the consequent potential for pathological change in another area of the body.

Investigating the entire equine fascial system is a large undertaking, and hence this book focuses solely on an area of the body that has a significant role in load bearing and is particularly vulnerable to overuse injuries and catastrophic breakdowns- that is, the forelimb. Although the primary focus of this book is the fascial connectivity in the forelimb, the significance of this cannot be grasped without a solid understanding of the already-described musculoskeletal elements of the forelimb. Hence, before diving into the fascial anatomy, a brief summary of the forelimb skeleton and muscles is presented. It is hoped that, together with this existing knowledge, the fascial anatomy presented in this book will help to further the current understanding of overall forelimb biomechanics and the development of compensatory postures and movement patterns which may occur with limb lameness and injury.

REFERENCES

Gehlsen, G., Ganion, L., & Helfst, R. (1991). Fibroblast responses to variation in soft tissue mobilization pressure. *Medicine and Science in Sports and Exercise, 31*, 531–535.

Hukins, D., & Aspden, R. (1985). Composition and properties of connective tissues. *Trends in Biochemical Sciences, 10*(7), 260–264.

Stecco, C. (2015). *Functional Atlas of the Human Fascial System*. Edinburgh: Elsevier.

BIBLIOGRAPHY

Alberts, B., Johnson, A., & Lewis, J. (2002). *Molecular Biology of the Cell* (4th ed.). New York, NY: Garland Science.

Barone, R. (2010). *Arthrologie et Myologie* (4th ed., Vol. 2). Paris: Éditions Vigot.

Baxter, G. (2011). *Adams and Stashak's Lameness in Horses* (G. Baxter, Ed., 6th ed., Revised ed.). Chichester: John Wiley & Sons.

Blasi, M., Blasi, J., Miguel-Pérez, M., Domingo, T., Dorca, E., García, M., & Pérez, A. (2012). Anatomical and histological study of fetus fascias. *Journal of Bodywork and Movement Therapies, 16*(4), 523.

Bradley, O. (1920). *The Topographical Anatomy of the Limbs of the Horse*. Edinburgh: W. Green & Son.

Caggiati, A. (2000). Fascial relations and structure of the tributaries of the saphenous veins. *Surgical and Radiologic Anatomy, 22*, 191–196.

Chauveau, A. (1873). *The Comparative Anatomy of the Domesticated Animals* (G. Fleming, Ed., 2nd ed.). New York, NY: D. Appleton and Company.

Chila, A. (2010). *Foundations of Osteopathic Medicine* (Revised ed.). Philadelphia, PA: Lippincott Williams & Wilkins.

DiGiovanna, E., Schiowitz, S., & Dowling, D. (2004). *An Osteopathic Approach to Diagnosis and Treatment* (Revised ed.). Philadelphia, PA: Lippincott Williams & Wilkins.

Egerbacher, M., Forstenpointer, G., Weissengruber, G., Licka, T., & Peham, C. (2012). Passive load-relevant structures of the musculoskeletal system in the forelimb of the horse. *Journal of Bodywork and Movement Therapies, 16*(3), 404–405.

Eichbaum, F. (1883). Fascien des Pferdes. *Archiv für die wissenschaftliche und praktische Tierheilkunde 14*, 280–308.

Gersh, I., & Catchpole, H. (1960). The nature of ground substance of connective tissue. *Perspectives in Biology and Medicine, 3*(2), 282–319.

International Committee on Veterinary Gross Anatomical Nomenclature. (2012). *Nomina Anatomica Veterinaria*. Hannover: Editorial Committee.

Jeffcott, L., Rossdale, P., Freestone, J., Frank, C., & Towers-Clark, P. (1982). An assessment of wastage in Thoroughbred racing from conception to 4 years of age. *Equine Veterinary Journal, 14*(3), 185–198.

Kawamata, S., Ozawa, J., Hashimoto, M., Kurose, T., & Shinohara, H. (2003). Structure of the rat subcutaneous connective tissue in relation to its sliding mechanism. *Archives of Histology and Cytology, 66*(3), 273–279.

Lindsay, M., & Robertson, C. (2008). *Fascia: Clinical Applications for Health and Human Performance*. New York, NY: Delmar Cengage Learning.

Myers, T. (2009). *Anatomy Trains: Myofascial Meridians for Manual and Movement Therapists* (2nd ed.). New York, NY: Elsevier.

Nickel, R., Schummer, A., Seiferle, E., Wilkens, H., Wille, K.-H., & Frewein, J. (1986). *The Anatomy of the Domestic Mammals* (Vol. 1). Berlin: Verlag Paul Parey.

Paulli, S., & Sörensen, E. (1930). *Die Fascien des Pferdes*. Kopenhagen, Dänemark: Königl Tierärytliche und Landwirtschaftliche Hochschule.

Porter, K., & Tucker, J. (1981). The ground substance of the living cell. *Scientific American, 244*(3), 56–67.

Schleip, R., Jäger, H., & Klinger, W. (2012). What is 'fascia'? A review of different nomenclatures. *Journal of Bodywork and Movement Therapies, 16*, 496–502.

Sisson, S., & Grossman, J. (1938). *The Anatomy of the Domestic Animals* (3rd ed.). Philadelphia, PA: W.B. Saunders.

Standring, S. (2008). *The Anatomical Basis of Clinical Practice* (40th ed.). Edinburgh: Elsevier Churchill Livingstone.

Stecco, C., Macchi, V., Porzionato, A., Duparc, F., & De Caro, R. (2011). The fascia: The forgotten structure. *Italian Journal of Anatomy and Embryology, 116*(3), 127–138.

van der Wal, J. (2009). The architecture of the connective tissue in the musculoskeletal system—an often overlooked functional parameter as to proprioception in the locomotor apparatus. *International Journal of Therapeutic Massage and Bodywork, 2*(4), 9–23.

CHAPTER 2

ANATOMY OF THE EQUINE FORELIMB

THE PROXIMAL FORELIMB

The equine forelimb, or thoracic limb, forms no direct articulation with the trunk and is instead supported in position via a musculature sling. The muscles comprising this sling include the trapezius, rhomboideus, latissimus dorsi, brachiocephalicus, serratus ventralis and the pectorals (superficial and deep). Details of their attachments are illustrated and described in *Table 2.1*. Hence, the most proximal bony articulation of the equine forelimb is the gleno-humeral (shoulder) joint (**Fig. 2.1**), which is comprised of the spherical head of the humerus articulating with the glenoid cavity of the scapula. The shoulder joint generally functions as a hinge joint which only allows for flexion and extension in the sagittal plane. Movement in the transverse plane is restricted by both a decreased convexity of the humeral head and by the attachment and relationships of the tendons of origin and insertion of surrounding muscles. These muscles are more or less arranged in medial and lateral groups but they enclose the shoulder joint on all sides.

Muscles situated on the lateral aspect of the shoulder region include the supraspinatus, infraspi-natus, deltoideus and teres minor, whilst those on the medial aspect include the subscapularis, teres major, articularis humeri and the coracobrachialis. The main function of each of these muscles is summarised in *Table 2.2*. The movements of the shoulder are also somewhat damped and limited by the connections and associations of the thick pad of fibrocartilage that lies within the tendon of origin of biceps brachii where it crosses the greater trochanter of the humerus. The bicipital bursa forms at this point where the fibrocartilage fits snugly over the sagittal ridge of the intertubercular groove thus limiting medial and lateral movements of the shoulder. The supraspinatus muscle has a particularly important role in the stabilisation of the joint. Together with the insertion of the super-ficial pectoral muscle, it limits abduction of the joint. In contrast, the infraspinatus muscle acts to prevent adduction of the shoulder joint and assists with shoulder joint flexion and extension. It has been said that ligaments which would otherwise act to support the joint in addition to the tendons of these muscles are absent at the shoulder joint. However, medial and lateral glenohumeral liga-ments which reinforce the joint capsule are often described.

Table 2.1 **Musculature of the equine pectoral girdle**

	MUSCLE	ORIGIN	INSERTION
Superficial layer	Trapezius 1. Cervicis 2. Thoracis	1. Funicular part of nuchal ligament from the second to third cervical vertebrae 2. Supraspinatus ligament from the third cervical to the tenth thoracic vertebrae	1. Spine of scapula 2. Aponeurotic insertion on upper third of scapula spine and fuses with shoulder fascia
	Sternomandibularis	Manubrium of the sternum	Sternomandibular tuberosity of the mandible
	Brachiocephalicus 1. Cleidomastoideus 2. Cleidobrachialis	1. Mastoid process of temporal bone and the nuchal crest 2. Clavicular tendon	1. Clavicular tendon 2. Deltoid tuberosity and crest of the humerus as well as fascia of the shoulder and arm
	Omotransversarius	Fascia of lateral shoulder region	Second to fourth cervical transverse processes
	Latissimus dorsi	Supraspinous ligament (from third thoracic to last lumbar vertebra) and thoracolumbar fascia	Medial aspect of the teres tubercle of the humerus
	Superficial pectoral 1. Descending pectoral 2. Transverse pectoral	1. Manubrium of the sternum 2. Sternum (between the 1st and 6th costal cartilages)	1. Brachial fascia and crest of the humerus 2. Antebrachial fascia
Deep layer	Deep pectoral 1. Subclavius (pars prescapularis) 2. Ascending pectoral (pars humeralis)	1. Sternum from the 1st to 4th costal cartilages 2. Sternum, costal cartilages of the 4th to 9th ribs and partly the tunica flava	1. Epimysium of cervical border of supraspinatus and lateral tuberosity of the humerus 2. Medial tuberosity of the humerus and tendon of origin of biceps brachii m. as well as lateral tuberosity of humerus
	Rhomboideus 1. Cervicis 2. Thoracis	1. Funicular part of the nuchal ligament from the level of the 2nd cervical to 2nd thoracic vertebra 2. Supraspinous ligament from the level of the 2nd to 8th thoracic vertebra	Both insert on the medial surface of the scapular cartilage
	Serratus ventralis 1. Cervicis 2. Thoracis	1. Transverse processes of 4th to 7th cervical vertebrae 2. Middle third of first 8–9 ribs and continuous with tunica flava. Deep surface unites with the superficial lamina of the spinocostotransverse fascia	Both attach to the serrated face of the scapula and the medial surface of the scapular cartilage

Source: Bradley, O., *The Topographical Anatomy of the Limbs of the Horse,* W. Green & Son, Edinburgh, 1920; Dyce, K. et al., *Textbook of Veterinary Anatomy,* 3rd ed., W.B. Saunders, Philadelphia, PA, 2002; Nickel, R. et al., *The Anatomy of the Domestic Mammals,* Vol. 1, Verlag Paul Parey, Berlin, 1986; Sisson, S., and Grossman, J., *The Anatomy of the Domestic Animals,* 3rd ed., W.B. Saunders, 1938.

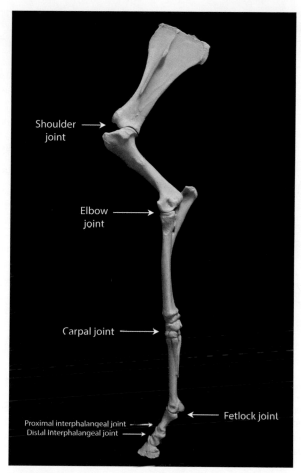

Fig. 2.1 **Skeleton of the left equine forelimb (lateral aspect).**

Distal to the shoulder joint is the elbow joint, which is formed by the articulation between three bones: the humerus, ulna and radius (**Figs. 2.1** and **2.2**). The elbow joint is slightly more complex than the shoulder joint in that it comprises two articular regions. These are the humeroradial articulation (between the distal extremity of the humerus and proximal extremity of the radius) and the humeroulnar articulation (between the distal extremity of the humerus and proximal extremity of the ulna).

The elbow joint is supported by strong collateral ligaments, which prevent lateral movement of the joint and make it a true ginglymus (hinge) joint. Collectively the attachments of the collateral ligaments subclassify the joint as a snap joint, capable of moving abruptly from a stable to mobile position. It has two positions of relative stability, one when fully flexed and the other when fully extended.

Table 2.2 **Musculature of the shoulder joint**

	MUSCLE	ORIGIN	INSERTION
Lateral aspect	Supraspinatus	Scapula cartilage; supraspinous fossa, cranial border and spine of the scapula	Greater and lesser tubercles of the humerus
	Infraspinatus	Scapula cartilage; infraspinous fossa; scapular spine	Directly to the free border of the greater tubercle of the humerus and via a separate tendon to a region immediately distal to the greater tubercle
	Deltoideus	Caudal border and spine of the scapula, as well as aponeurosis of infraspinatus	Deltoid tuberosity and the brachial fascia
	Teres minor	Distal half of caudal border of scapula	Teres minor tuberosity proximal to the deltoid tuberosity
Medial aspect	Subscapularis	Subscapular fossa	Lesser tubercle of the humerus and shoulder joint capsule
	Teres major	Dorsal angle and caudal border of the scapula and subscapular muscle	Teres major tuberosity after joining with the tendon of the latissimus dorsi
	Articularis humeri	Scapula immediately proximal to the margin of the glenoid fossa	Neck of the humerus
	Coracobrachialis	Coracoid process of scapula	Craniomedial surface of humerus distal to the teres major tuberosity

Source: Bradley, O., *The Topographical Anatomy of the Limbs of the Horse*, W. Green & Son, Edinburgh, 1920; Dyce, K. et al., *Textbook of Veterinary Anatomy*, 3rd ed., W.B. Saunders, Philadelphia, PA, 2002; Nickel, R. et al., *The Anatomy of the Domestic Mammals*, Vol. 1, Verlag Paul Parey, Berlin, 1986; Sisson, S., and Grossman, J., *The Anatomy of the Domestic Animals*, 3rd ed., W.B. Saunders, 1938.

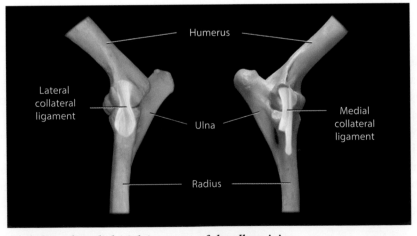

Fig. 2.2 Lateral (left) and medial (right) aspects of the elbow joint.

Table 2.3 **Musculature of the elbow joint**

MUSCLE	ORIGIN	INSERTION
Biceps brachii	Supraglenoid tubercle of scapula	(1) Radial tuberosity, (2) proximal border of the radius and (3) antebrachial fascia and extensor carpi radialis muscle via the lacertus fibrosis
Brachialis	Humerus neck and caudal surface	Medial aspect of the radius distal to the biceps tendon
Triceps brachii 1. Long head 2. Lateral head 3. Medial head	1. Caudal border of the scapula 2. Tricipital line and brachial fascia 3. Medial surface of the distal half of the humerus	1. Olecranon of ulna 2. Lateral aspect of olecranon and partly with the tendon of the long head 3. Medial surface of the olecranon
Anconeus	Distal half of the caudal border of the humerus and the lateral and medial epicondyles	Lateral aspect of the olecranon (partly attached to the proximal diverticulum of the joint capsule)
Tensor fasciae antebrachii	Caudal border of the scapula and terminal tendon of latissimus dorsi	Antebrachial fascia and the medial surface of the olecranon

Source: Bradley, O., *The Topographical Anatomy of the Limbs of the Horse*, W. Green & Son, Edinburgh, 1920; Dyce, K. et al., *Textbook of Veterinary Anatomy*, 3rd ed., W.B. Saunders, Philadelphia, PA, 2002; Nickel, R. et al., *The Anatomy of the Domestic Mammals*, Vol. 1, Verlag Paul Parey, Berlin, 1986; Sisson, S., and Grossman, J., *The Anatomy of the Domestic Animals*, 3rd ed., W.B. Saunders, 1938.

The muscles surrounding the radius and ulna distal to the elbow joint in the antebrachium are summarised and illustrated in *Table 2.3* and **Figs. 2.2–2.4** respectively. Their tendons of insertions either attach to the bones comprising the carpus or to the bones comprising the distal portion of the forelimb. The carpus itself is comprised of three joints including the antebrachiocarpal joint (formed between the distal extremity of the radius and the proximal row of carpal bones), the middle carpal joint (formed between the two rows of carpal bones) and the carpometacarpal joint (formed between the distal row of carpal bones and the proximal extremity of the metacarpal bones) (*Table 2.4*).

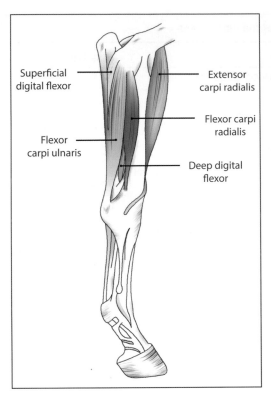

Fig. 2.3 Musculature of the antebrachium (medial aspect).

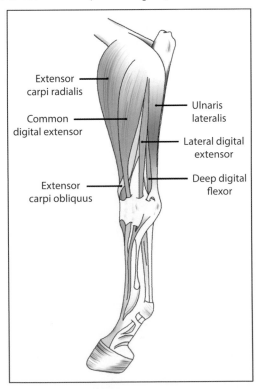

Fig. 2.4 Musculature of the antebrachium (lateral aspect).

Table 2.4 **Musculature of the carpal joint and digit**

	MUSCLE	ORIGIN	INSERTION
Extensor muscles	Extensor carpi radialis	Crest of the lateral epicondyle of the humerus, radial fossa and deltoid tuberosity	Metacarpal tuberosity
	Extensor carpi obliquus (abductor pollicis longus)	Lateral border of the cranial surface of the middle of the radius	Proximal extremity of the second metacarpal bone
	Common digital extensor	Proximal to the condyle of the humerus, lateral collateral ligament of the elbow joint and the cranial aspect of the lateral protuberance of the radius	Extensor process of the distal phalanx and the dorsal surfaces of the proximal extremities of the proximal and middle phalanx
	Lateral digital extensor	Lateral tuberosity of the radius and the lateral collateral ligament of the elbow joint, and the lateral border of the radius	Dorsolateral aspect of the proximal phalanx
Flexor muscles	Ulnaris lateralis (extensor carpi ulnaris)	Lateral epicondyle of the humerus	Accessory carpal bone
	Superficial digital flexor	Medial epicondyle of the humerus and posterior surface of the radius	The eminences on the proximal extremities of the middle phalanx and the distal extremity of the proximal phalanx
	Deep digital flexor	Medial epicondyle of the humerus, medial aspect of the olecranon and the middle of the caudal surface of the radius	Flexor surface of the distal phalanx
	Flexor carpi ulnaris	Medial epicondyle of the humerus (humeral head) and medial aspect of olecranon (ulnar head)	Accessory carpal bone
	Flexor carpi radialis	Medial epicondyle of the humerus	Proximal end of second metacarpal bone

Source: Bradley, O., *The Topographical Anatomy of the Limbs of the Horse*, W. Green & Son, Edinburgh, 1920; Dyce, K. et al., *Textbook of Veterinary Anatomy*, 3rd ed., W.B. Saunders, Philadelphia, PA, 2002; Nickel, R. et al., *The Anatomy of the Domestic Mammals*, Vol. 1, Verlag Paul Parey, Berlin, 1986; Sisson, S., and Grossman, J., *The Anatomy of the Domestic Animals*, 3rd ed., W.B. Saunders, 1938.

THE DISTAL FORELIMB

The distal forelimb is ultimately devoid of muscles and is instead propelled forward through the pull of tendons and ligaments that arise from muscles of the proximal forelimb and shoulder girdle. The skeleton of the equine distal forelimb (**Figs. 2.1** and **2.5**) is highly specialised in order to manage substantial loads and achieve high locomotory efficiency. The bones of this region represent a skeletal axis along which 55%–60% of the horse's entire body weight is distributed at rest (Dyce, Sack, & Wensing, 2002). These bones include the second, third and

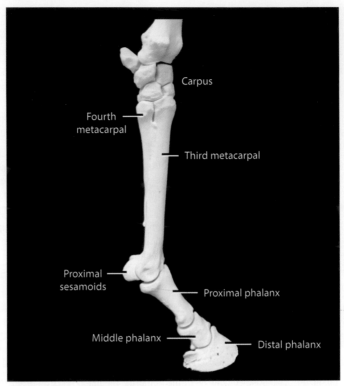

Fig. 2.5 Skeleton of the right distal forelimb (lateral aspect).

fourth metacarpals, the proximal, middle and distal phalanges, two proximal sesamoids bones (PSBs) and one distal sesamoid bone. Articulation between these bones, particularly the third metacarpal bone and phalanges, indicates how major forces are directed through the limb. Furthermore, the ligamentous and tendinous connections associated with the distal limb are an important aspect in the passive structural support of the limb.

The Mc3 is straight and robust and is thought to act as the primary weight-bearing bone in the distal forelimb. Clinically, it is subject to frequent injury (mostly fracture), particularly in horses subject to intense training and involved in high performance activities. On the mediopalmar and lateropalmar aspects of the Mc3, are the Mc2 and Mc4 respectively (colloquially known as the splint bones).

On the palmar surface of its distal extremity, the Mc3 articulates with the concaved articular surface of two PSBs. These are pyramidal shaped bones (connected to each other via fibrocartilage) which lie deep to the deep digital flexor tendon (DDFT). Distal to the metacarpus, the proximal, middle and distal phalanges form the skeleton of the third digit.

The distal extremity of Mc3, together with the proximal extremity of the PP, and both PSBs comprise the fetlock joint. Thus, the joint has two articulating surfaces: one between the distal extremity of Mc3 and the proximal extremity of the PP, and another between the distal palmar surface of the Mc3 and the concave surface of the two PSBs. A sagittal ridge divides the distal extremity of Mc3 into a medial and lateral surface. This conforms perfectly to the proximal extremity of the PP, which is similarly divided into a medial and lateral articular surface by a sagittal groove. The two PSBs lie either side of the sagittal ridge on the palmar side of the Mc3. These articulations, in addition to the collateral metacarpophalangeal and metacarposesamoidean ligaments either side of the joint (see below), allow for an extensive range of flexion and extension in the sagittal plane but only a minimal amount of rotation and lateral movement when in extension.

PASSIVE SUPPORT OF THE FORELIMB

When standing, the relative arrangement of the Mc3 and PP together with the direction of ground reaction forces acting on the limb, maintain the fetlock joint in a passive state of extension. Hyperextension of the joint is limited due to the passive resistance offered by the interosseous ligament, sesamoidean ligaments, and the digital flexor tendons associated with the joint. Together, these structures comprise passive support apparatuses including the suspensory apparatus (**Fig. 2.6**) and the passive stay apparatus. The suspensory apparatus (**Fig. 2.6**) prevents hyperextension of the fetlock joint and exists as a critical component of the passive stay apparatus, which provides passive resistance to flexion of other joints in the forelimb when under load. The digital flexors and their respective check (accessory) ligaments are commonly recognised as the major components of the stay apparatus in the distal portion of the forelimb.

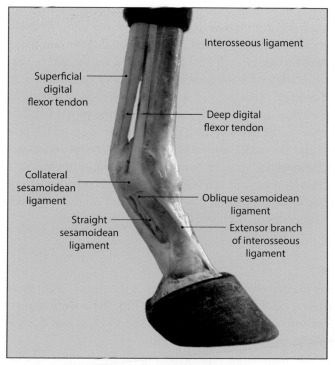

Fig. 2.6 **Suspensory apparatus in the equine distal forelimb.**

LIGAMENTS AND SOFT TISSUES OF THE DISTAL FORELIMB

Joint capsules

The metacarpophalangeal joint (MCPJ) has a spacious capsule, which is reinforced on the dorsal, medial and lateral aspects by tough fibrous bands. Extensive mobility of the joint is enabled via a dorsal and palmar pouch, both of which are important clinically as they can be easily penetrated from the medial and lateral aspects of the region immediately proximal to the joint and hence can reduce the risk of needle damage to the articular cartilage when injecting the joint or sampling the joint fluid.

The dorsal pouch lies under the common and lateral digital extensor tendons, which are further cushioned by a bursa in this location. The proximal boundary of this pouch forms a fold which projects distally into the centre of the pouch, and can result in lameness when inflamed. The palmar pouch is situated between the branches of the interosseous ligament and the distal extremity of the metacarpus.

Fused with the joint capsule on either side are the medial and lateral metacarpophalangeal collateral ligaments. Each of these arise as stout bands on the distal depressions of the Mc3 epicondyles and attach slightly distal to the articular margin of the proximal phalanx. As alluded to earlier, movement of the PP relative to the Mc3 is mostly constrained to the sagittal plane by these ligaments.

Sesamoidean ligaments

Several distal sesamoidean ligaments act in unison with each other in order to maintain the relative position of the PSBs and prevent extreme hyperflexion of the joint. These ligaments include the collateral, intersesamoidean, straight, paired oblique, paired short and paired cruciate sesamoidean ligaments. The axial surface of each PSB is connected via the intersesamoidean ligament and fibrocartilage, which still allows for independent function of each bone during movement of the MCPJ. The short and cruciate distal sesamoidean ligaments each attach the base of the PSBs to the proximopalmar margin of the proximal articular surface of the proximal phalanx. The straight sesamoidean ligament connects the bases of the PSBs to fibrocartilage on the proximal palmar margin of the middle phalanx, and the medial and lateral oblique sesamoidian ligaments course from their origins either side of the straight ligament to insert at an oblique angle onto the palmar surface of P1. A collateral sesamoidean ligament is also present on each side of the fetlock joint. They arise from the abaxial surface of each PSB and bifurcate to insert on depressions on the epicondyles of Mc3 and on proximal tubercles on both sides of the proximal phalanx.

Flexor tendons

The flexor tendons are located on the palmar aspect of the distal forelimb and include the superficial digital flexor tendon (SDFT) and the DDFT (**Fig. 2.7**). Both are situated on the palmar aspect of the distal forelimb and function to flex the fetlock joint and digit, as well as to store and release elastic strain energy throughout locomotion.

The SDFT is an extension of the superficial digital flexor muscle, which originates on the medial epicondyle of the humerus. The tendon becomes distinct at the level of the carpus, proximal to which it fuses with the narrow band of its proximal check (accessory) ligament that

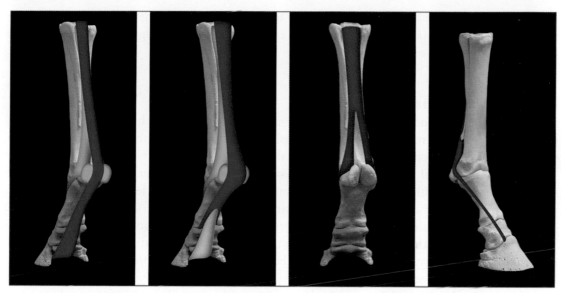

Fig. 2.7 Flexor tendons and ligaments of the distal forelimb (*from left to right: deep digital flexor tendon, superficial digital flexor tendon, interosseous ligament, extensor branch of interosseous ligament*). Distal ligaments of the proximal sesamoid bones are not shown.

originates on the distal medial border of the radius. The SDFT continues distally and envelops the DDFT at the level of the fetlock joint. At the approximate middle of the PP, it splits into two branches; however, the descriptions provided on where these branches insert is variable among authors. Generally, reports indicate that each of the branches inserts on the distal aspect of the PP as well as on the proximal aspect of the middle phalanx (Bradley, 1920; Dyce et al., 2002; Nickel et al., 1986; Sisson & Grossman, 1938; Zietzschmann, 1925). Other authors describe the SDFT branches to insert only on the proximal aspect of the middle phalanx (Barone, 2010; Share-Jones, 1907; Weaver, Stover, & O'Brien, 1992). It has been suggested that the branches that were perceived to insert on the distal end of the PP are in fact ligaments of the proximal interphalangeal joint (Weaver, Stover, & O'Brien, 1992). Authors who describe an SDFT branch insertion on the proximal phalanx only describe 2 pairs of proximal interphalangeal joint ligaments, which include the axial and superficial abaxial palmar ligaments. In contrast, authors reporting attachment of the SDFT branches only on the middle phalanx describe three pairs of proximal interphalangeal joint ligaments including an axial, superficial abaxial and a deep abaxial pair.

Descriptions provided for the DDFT are, in contrast, much more consistent. The DDFT arises from the three muscle bellies of the deep digital flexor muscle that originate on the medial epicondyle of the humerus and the caudal surfaces of the radius and ulna. The conjoined tendon continues distally along the dorsal (deep) aspect of the SDFT and ends at its insertion on the flexor surface of P3. It becomes easily palpable in the digit at the point where the SDFT separates into two branches. In the middle of the metacarpus, it is joined by the thick fibrous band of the distal check (accessory) ligament which arises from the palmar ligament of the carpus.

The interosseous ligament arises at the proximal end of the palmar aspect of the Mc3. It courses distally between the 2 splint bones and bifurcates proximal to the sesamoid bones (**Fig. 2.7**).

The two branches attach medially and laterally to the sesamoid bones before running obliquely and dorsally to join into the medial and lateral edges of the common digital extensor tendon in the region of the proximal phalanx.

Extensor tendons

The digital extensor tendons (**Fig. 2.8**) arise from muscles which lie on the dorsolateral aspect of the forearm. They are responsible for the extension of the distal forelimb joints and include the common digital extensor tendon and the lateral digital extensor tendon.

The common digital extensor tendon begins at the junction between the middle and distal thirds of the antebrachium where it arises from the like named muscle. It crosses the lateral aspect of the carpus then, as the tendon continues distally, it passes obliquely over the dorsolateral surface of the metacarpus and the dorsal surface of the PP and the middle phalanx. Thereafter, details on the common digital extensor tendon vary depending on the source. The majority of authors describe that it inserts on the proximal phalanx and/or the middle phalanx, in addition to having a major termination on the distal phalanx (Barone, 2010; Chauveau, 1873; Sisson & Grossman, 1938). A few authors have recognised some adherence of the tendon to the dorsum of the proximal phalanx via its attachment to the fascia which, in turn, attaches to the joint capsule (Nickel et al., 1986; Weaver, Stover, & O'Brien, 1992).

The lateral digital extensor tendon arises from the lateral digital extensor muscle situated on the lateral aspect of the antebrachium. It extends distally over the metacarpal bone lateral to the common digital extensor tendon. The tendon then crosses the fetlock joint and inserts on the dorsolateral aspect of the PP.

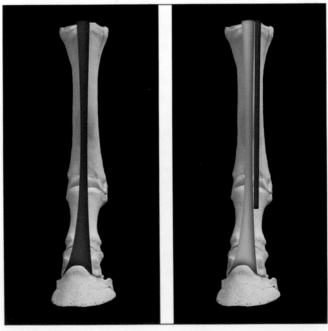

Fig. 2.8 Extensor tendons and ligaments of the distal forelimb (*left: common digital extensor tendon; right: lateral digital extensor tendon*).

Annular ligaments

On the palmar aspect of the fetlock joint and pastern region, there are three annular ligaments described as being responsible for holding the flexor tendons in place. The palmar annular ligament has an attachment from the SDFT to the abaxial border of the PSBs. The proximal digital annular ligament also blends with the SDFT. It lies distal to the palmar annular ligament and resembles an X shape. Its four corners attach to the medial and lateral borders of the proximal phalanx. The distal annular ligament extends from the proximal to the distal phalanx between the DDFT and digital cushion.

REFERENCES

Barone, R. (2010). *Arthrologie et Myologie* (4th ed., Vol. 2). Paris: Éditions Vigot.

Chauveau, A. (1873). *The Comparative Anatomy of the Domesticated Animals* (G. Fleming, Ed., 2nd ed.). New York, NY: D. Appleton and Company.

Dyce, K., Sack, W., & Wensing, C. (2002). *Textbook of Veterinary Anatomy* (3rd ed.). Philadelphia, PA: W.B. Saunders.

Nickel, R., Schummer, A., Seiferle, E., Wilkens, H., Wille, K.-H., & Frewein, J. (1986). *The Anatomy of the Domestic Mammals* (Vol. 1). Berlin: Verlag Paul Parey.

Share-Jones, J. (1907). *The Surgical Anatomy of the Horse Part II.- Fore Limb*. New York, NY: William R. Jenkins Co.

Sisson, S., & Grossman, J. (1938). *The Anatomy of the Domestic Animals* (3rd ed.). Philadelphia, PA: W.B. Saunders.

Weaver, J., Stover, S. M., & O'Brien, T. (1992). Radiographic anatomy of soft tissue attachments in the equine metacarpophalangeal and proximal phalangeal region. *Equine Veterinary Journal, 24*(4), 310–315.

Zietzschmann, O. (1925). *Spezielle Bewegungslehre*. Berlin.

BIBLIOGRAPHY

Alexander, G., Gibson, K., Day, R., & Robertson, I. (2001). Effects of superior check desmotomy on flexor tendon and suspensory ligament strain in equine cadaver limbs. *Veterinary Surgery, 30*, 522–527.

Bailey, C. (1998). *Wastage in the Australian Thoroughbred Industry*. Retrieved from http://www.hestefor-skning.com/wp-content/uploads/2015/05/Wastage-Australia.pdf.

Baxter, G. (2011). *Adams and Stashak's Lameness in Horses* (G. Baxter, Ed., 6th ed., Revised ed.). Chichester: John Wiley & Sons.

Biewener, A., Thomason, J., & Lanyon, L. (1983). Mechanics of locomotion and jumping in the forelimb of the horse (Equus): In vivo stress developed in the radius and metacarpus. *Journal of Zoology, 201*(1), 67–82. doi:10.1111/j.1469-7998.1983.tb04261.x

Bradley, O. (1920). *The Topographical Anatomy of the Limbs of the Horse*. Edinburgh: W. Green & Son.

Brama, P., Karssenberg, D., Barneveld, A., & van Weeren, P. (2001). Contact areas and pressure distribution on the proximal articular surface of the proximal phalanx under sagittal plane loading. *Equine Veterinary Journal, 33*(1), 26–32.

Budras, K.-D., Sack, W. O., & Röck, S. (2003). *Anatomy of the Horse: An Illustrated Text* (4th ed.). Hannover: Schlütersche.

Davies, H., Philip, C., & Merritt, J. (2007). Chapter 2- Functional anatomy of the equine digit: Determining function from structure. In A. Floyd & R. Mansmann (Eds.), *Equine Podiatry* (pp. 25–41). London: Elsevier Health Sciences.

Estberg, L., Stover, S., Gardner, I., Johnson, B., Case, J., Ardans, A., … Woods, L. (1996). Fatal musculo-skeletal injuries incurred during racing and training in thoroughbreds. *Journal of the American Veterinary Medical Association, 208*(1), 92–96.

Ferraro, G., Stover, S., & Whitcomb, M. (2007). *Suspensory Ligament Injuries in Horses.* Davis, CA: Centre for Equine Health, University of California.

Getman, L., Sutter, W., & Bertone, A. (2014). Infections of muscle, joint, and bone. In D. Sellon & M. Long (Eds.), *Equine Infectious Diseases* (2nd ed., pp. 60–70). St. Louis, MO: Saunders Elsevier.

Gibson, K., & Steel, C. (2002). Conditions of the suspensory ligament causing lameness in horses. *Equine Veterinary Education, 14,* 39–50.

Hernandez, J., Hawkins, D., & Scollay, M. (2001). Race-start characteristics and risk of catastrophic mus-culoskeletal injury in Thoroughbred racehorses. *Journal of the American Veterinary Medical Association, 218*(1), 83–86.

Hill, A., Gardner, I., Carpenter, T., & Stover, S. (2004). Effects of injury to the suspensory apparatus, exercise, and horseshoe characteristics on the risk of lateral condylar fracture and suspensory apparatus failure in forelimbs of Thoroughbred racehorses. *American Journal of Veterinary Research, 65,* 1508.

Hubert, J., Latimer, F., & Moore, R. (2001). Proximal sesamoid bone fractures in horses. *The Compendium on Continuing Education for the Practicing Veterinarian, 23*(7), 678–687.

Kane, A., Stover, S., Gardner, I., Case, J., Johnson, B., Read, D., & Ardans, A. (1996). Horseshoe charac-teristics as possible risk factors for fatal musculoskeletal injury of Thoroughbred racehorses. *American Journal of Veterinary Research, 57,* 1147–1152.

König, H., Liebich, H., & Bragulla, H. (2007). *Veterinary Anatomy of Domestic Mammals: Textbook and Colour Atlas.* Stuttgart: Schattauer.

McIlwraith, C., Frisbie, D., & Kawcak, C. (2001). Current treatments for traumatic synovitis, capsulitis, and osteoarthritis. *Proceedings of the American Association of Equine Practitioners, 47,* 180–206.

McKerney, E., Collar, E., & Stover, S. (2013). Fatal musculoskeletal injuries of the metacarpophalangeal and metatarsophalangeal (fetlock) joints in California racehorses: One hundred thirty-nine cases. *Paper presented at the Proceedings of the 59th Annual Convention of the American Association of Equine Practitioners,* Nashville, TN.

Peloso, J., Mundy, G., & Cohen, N. (1994). Prevalence of, and factors associated with, musculoskeletal rac-ing injuries of thoroughbreds. *Journal of the American Veterinary Medical Association, 204,* 620–626.

Pilliner, S., & Davies, Z. (2004). *Equine Science* (2nd ed.). Oxford: Blackwell Publishing.

Pollitt, C. (2015). *The Illustrated Horse's Foot: A Comprehensive Guide.* London: Elsevier Health Sciences.

Ross, M., & Dyson, S. (2010). *Diagnosis and Management of Lameness in the Horse.* Philadelphia, PA: W.B. Saunders.

Sisson, S., Grossman, J., & Getty, R. (1975). *Sisson and Grossman's the Anatomy of the Domestic Animals.* Philadelphia, PA: W.B. Saunders.

Stashak, T., & Adams, O. (2002). *Adams' Lameness in Horses.* Philadelphia, PA: Lippincott Williams & Wilkins.

Vanderperren, K., & Saunders, J. (2009a). Diagnostic imaging of the equine fetlock region using radiog-raphy and ultrasonography. Part 1: Soft tissues. *The Veterinary Journal, 181,* 111–122.

Vanderperren, K., & Saunders, J. (2009b). Diagnostic imaging of the equine fetlock region using radiogra-phy. Part 2: The bony disorders. *The Veterinary Journal, 181,* 123–136.

Wilson, A., McGuigan, M., Su, A., & van den Bogert, A. (2001). Horses damp the spring in their step. *Nature, 414,* 895–899.

Wilson, A., Watson, J., & Lichtwark, G. (2003). Biomechanics: A catapult action for rapid limb protraction. *Nature, 421*(6918), 35–36.

INTRODUCTION

The equine distal forelimb has a highly specialised anatomical design, which allows for a high degree of locomotory efficiency and speed. Its contribution to the overall proficiency of locomotion in the horse is achieved via a passive energy storage and release system that enables longstanding support and rapid limb protraction with minimal muscular expenditure.

Compliant tendons of the superficial and deep digital flexor muscles, as well as the collagenous interosseous muscle, allow for the passive storage and return of elastic energy throughout locomotion. Dorsiflexion of the metacarpophalangeal joint stretches these structures, which span most, if not the entire length, of the distal forelimb. Consequently, the superficial digital flexor tendon (SDFT), deep digital flexor tendon (DDFT) and interosseous ligament are subject to large changes in length when under load (8%–12% strain or approximately 7 cm elongation in an average 70 cm tendon).

Because of this anatomical design, these structures are particularly vulnerable to overuse injuries and catastrophic breakdown. In fact, structures comprising the distal forelimb are involved in almost half of all reported forelimb musculoskeletal injuries, which themselves contribute the largest percentage of recognised injuries in racing and performance horses.

An understanding of the aetiology and management of such frequently occurring pathologies in the distal forelimb is largely dependent on a thorough understanding of the distal forelimb functional anatomy and support mechanisms. The current literature surrounding these areas is limited in that it describes discrete, often functionally isolated, anatomical structures and fails to consider the connective tissue, or fascial expansions, functionally and mechanically integrating these structures. As a consequence, there remain gaps in the fundamental understanding of forelimb loading patterns and the inherent stabilising mechanisms, which support the joints of the distal limbs.

The significance of the mechanical linkages provided by the fascia is a concept that is slowly beginning to filter into the literature. Studies have found that mechanical reactions to landing in the human leg, caused by tensional distribution throughout the body's linked segments, contribute to physical adjustments more rapidly than neural reflex mechanisms. These types of mechanical reactions have not previously been considered in the field of equine biomechanics, yet they provide an effective solution to responding to ground perturbations during rapid locomotion when neural reflex mechanisms may be too slow to stimulate a change.

It is this emerging research which has inspired this anatomic investigation into the fascia of the equine forelimb. Research focusing on the significance of fascia in equine forelimb biomechanics is noticeably lacking in the literature, yet analysis of simple fascial characteristics, such as attachment points, fibre direction and thickness, can be directly informative of the paths of load distribution and areas subject to most strain. Such knowledge has the potential to greatly improve the current understanding of equine forelimb kinematics and loading, and to provide a basis for further study of the fascial system in the horse.

SUPERFICIAL FASCIA

General findings

A superficial fascial layer identified over the metacarpus, fetlock and proximal digit, is continuous proximally with the superficial fascia of the carpus and antebrachium (**Fig. 3.1**). It appears macroscopically to consist of two delicate sheets, which are not readily separated in any of the specimens dissected. On gross observation, both sheets have a highly irregular and unspecialised arrangement of collagen fibres, which align according to the direction of tension applied.

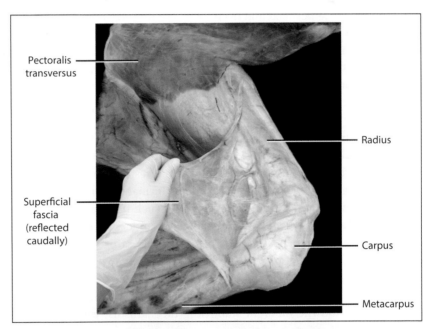

Fig. 3.1 **Medial aspect of left antebrachium, carpus, and proximal metacarpus.**

The functional significance of fascial layers

The superficial fascia can be clearly detached from the overlying skin and the underlying deep fascia in some regions, and yet fuses strongly to either or both in other regions, suggesting that it has a role in both the functional isolation of tissue planes as well as in the support of subcutaneous structures. In areas where it is clearly separable as a defined membrane (palmar, dorsal and dorsomedial aspect of the metacarpus), it allows sliding to occur between the skin and the underlying structures- a role most likely achieved via the lubricating role of the ground substance (Stecco, 2015) comprising the loose connective tissue located between the superficial fascia and both the overlying subcutaneous tissue and the underlying deep fascia. In contrast, areas where the superficial fascia attaches to either the subcutis or the deep fascia suggests that it is important in supporting and maintaining the position of the skin and underlying structures, as well as in directing and distributing tension.

In the region of the metacarpus (Mc3), the superficial fascia exists as a relatively elastic medium between the skin and underlying structures. Its attachment to the skin over most of the distal forelimb is via loose connective tissue which allows for relatively easy separation of the two layers. This, in addition to its fluidic consistency, permits a small amount of gliding between the tissue planes over the metacarpal region. Distal to the fetlock joint, the superficial fascia becomes a much tighter and inelastic support sheet for the structures of the proximal digit and is more tightly adhered to the overlying skin.

Dorsal, medial and lateral aspects

On the dorsal aspect, the superficial fascia can be peeled away from the underlying fascia enveloping the extensor tendons along most of their length. It thins distal to the metacarpophalangeal joint (MCPJ) and, with careful dissection, can be followed to a short distance (approximately 1 cm) above the hoof capsule (**Figs. 3.2** and **3.3**). In the proximal two-thirds of the Mc3, the superficial fascia continues around the medial to palmar aspects, remaining as a distinct layer superficial to the deeper fascial layers comprising and extending from the flexor tendon sheath (**Fig. 3.4**). Laterally, the superficial fascia merges with the underlying deep fascia along the lateral border of the lateral digital extensor tendon (LDET). This fusion extends from immediately distal to a band of fascia connecting the accessory carpal bone to the LDET, to the approximate level of the distal end of the fourth metacarpal bone (Mc4) (**Fig. 3.5**). Together, the merged layers continue around the lateral and palmar aspects of the proximal two-thirds of the Mc3, and join with the continuation of the superficial fascia extending from the medial aspect.

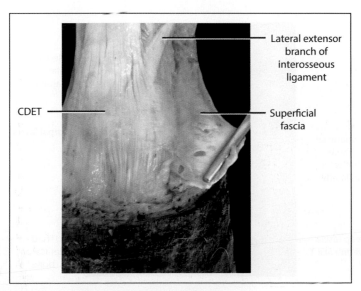

Fig. 3.2 Superficial fascia over the dorsal aspect of left digit.

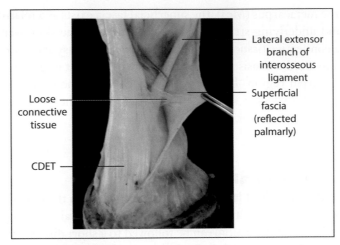

Fig. 3.3 Dorsolateral aspect of the digit.

Cross-hatching in the carpal tendon sheath

The characteristic cross-hatched arrangement of collagen fibres in the distal extension of the carpal fascia is necessary for the overall support and stability of the joint. Such an arrangement of fibrils is commonly adopted in nature and in the manufacturing of materials. Secondary plant cell walls for example have cross-hatched layering of microfibrils which ensures overall strength of the wall and still allows for longitudinal growth (Bowsher, Steer, & Tobin, 2008). The same principle is used in the manufacture of fibreglass-epoxy structures such as fishing rods and planes where great strength for weight is essential (Smith, 1977). On the palmar aspect of the carpus and proximal metacarpus, such a design provides a directed path for load distribution and provides mechanically efficient resistance to flexor tendon and carpal joint movement. This role is enforced via its attachment and continuation over the splint bones as well as through its expansion across the superficial surface of the interosseous ligament (IL). Its connection to the IL may aid in the transfer of strain through the carpus and to structures in the antebrachium, so that loads propagated through the IL are not concentrated at its point of origin at the proximal margin of the Mc3.

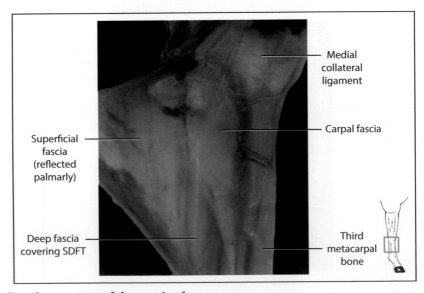

Fig. 3.4 Mediopalmar aspect of the proximal metacarpus.

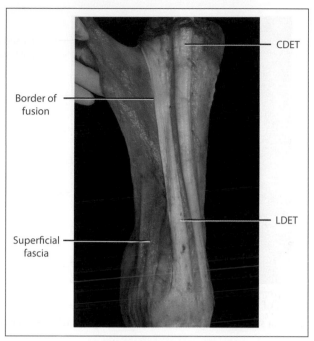

Fig. 3.5 Fusion of the superficial and deep fascial layers along the lateral border of the lateral digital extensor tendon.

Fascial layers and their role in load bearing

The superficial fascia thins and becomes difficult to separate as a distinct layer by the level of the proximal interphalangeal joint and this may reflect the stability required from the CDET and the extensor branches of the IL in order to support the digit and manage impact related force and strain.

The fusion between fascial layers on the dorsal aspect of the metacarpus, along the lateral border of the LDET correlates with the normal pattern of forelimb loading in the horse. During the stance phase, horses tend to land first on the lateral aspect of the hoof and then preferentially load the medial side of the forelimb. Therefore, fusion of the superficial and deep fascia dorsolaterally along the LDET may assist, in a small way, in maintaining the stability and overall balance of the distal forelimb in response to forces propagated at or immediately after impact. Rather than tension being concentrated on either the superficial or deep fascial layer, fusion between the superficial and deep fascial layers allows for an increased surface area over which tensional forces can be distributed and promotes a line of increased strength and rigidity.

In contrast, the lack of fusion over the dorsomedial aspect possibly allows for the transfer of tensile forces medially throughout the stance phase to increase the likelihood of an even distribution of load throughout the metacarpal region. This may occur via the interaction of ground substance molecules comprising the loose connective tissue between the superficial and deep fascial layers. Fluid mechanics suggests that a net force applied to liquid will cause it to flow in the direction of least pressure due to its lack of rigidity. As the ground substance of loose connective tissue follows the laws of fluid mechanics, this suggests that a medial transfer of load in the metacarpus is enabled via a pressure imbalance created laterally at ground impact, which then causes medial flow of ground substance molecules in order to reach pressure equilibrium.

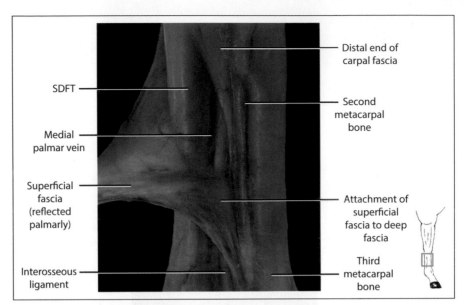

Fig. 3.6 Mediopalmar aspect of the left mid-shaft metacarpus. Note the connectivity between the superficial fascia and the fascia surrounding the interosseous ligament, the medial palmar nerve and vessels.

SDFT changes of length

In the distal half of the metacarpus the deep fascia extending proximally from the ergot tissue divides into two thin layers over the surface of the SDFT. In addition to the superficial fascia, these layers provide a lubricating medium between the skin and SDFT (Guimberteau, Delage, & Wong, 2010). Being on the flexor aspect of the distal forelimb, the SDFT undergoes a substantial increase in length with fetlock hyperflexion. As the skin is anchored to the palmar annular ligament of the fetlock joint via the ergot tissue, the same degree of vertical stretch in the skin is not observed. Therefore, the fascial layers between the skin and SDFT most likely allow for a necessary degree of functional and mechanical isolation of the SDFT from the skin throughout locomotion.

In the distal third of the Mc3, the superficial fascia extending around the medial and lateral aspects forms a fascial hiatus that intricately arranges around the palmar vessels and nerves running alongside the flexor tendons. Through this hiatus, the superficial fascia becomes connected to the deep fascia surrounding and investing between the flexor tendons on the palmar aspect (**Figs. 3.6–3.8**).

In the region of the fetlock joint, the superficial fascia is more strongly connected to the underlying fascia on the dorsal aspect over the juncture between the common digital extensor tendon (CDET) and the LDET. It can, however, still be separated away as a distinct layer. As described earlier, it thins over the surface of the CDET as it approaches the hoof capsule and becomes inseparable from this tendon a short distance proximal to the coronary band of the hoof capsule (**Figs. 3.2** and **3.3**).

On the medio- and latero-dorsal aspects of the proximal phalanx, fibrous connective tissue attaches the superficial fascia to the deep fascia in the region proximal to where the CDET and the extensor branches of the IL meet (**Fig. 3.9**). Fusion between the superficial and deep fascia is also observed palmar to the extensor branches of the interosseous ligament (**Figs. 3.10** and **3.11**).

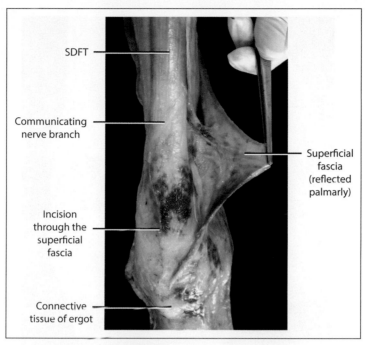

SDFT

Communicating
nerve branch

Incision
through the
superficial
fascia

Connective
tissue of ergot

Superficial
fascia
(reflected
palmarly)

Fig. 3.7 Palmar aspect of the left metacarpus.

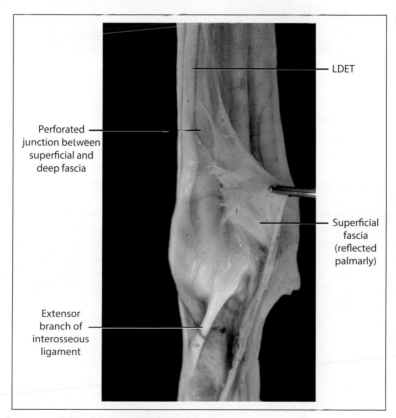

LDET

Perforated
junction between
superficial and
deep fascia

Extensor
branch of
interosseous
ligament

Superficial
fascia
(reflected
palmarly)

Fig. 3.8 Lateral aspect of distal half of the left metacarpus and metacarpophalangeal joint.

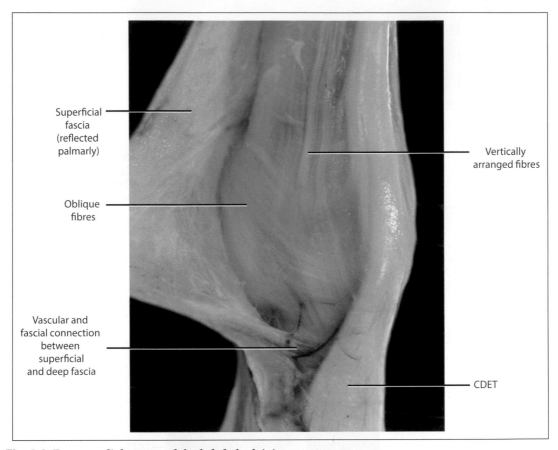

Superficial fascia (reflected palmarly)

Oblique fibres

Vascular and fascial connection between superficial and deep fascia

Vertically arranged fibres

CDET

Fig. 3.9 Dorsomedial aspect of the left fetlock joint.

Fascial bands of the distal forelimb

The deep fascia extending between the CDET and IL extensor branches is likely to have a role in functionally integrating these two structures. Distally, the extensor branches run an oblique course across the fetlock to unite with the CDET on the dorsal aspect of the proximal phalanx. Therefore, it is likely that the vertical and oblique orientation of collagen fibres, that is grossly evident in the fascia extending between the extensor tendons and the IL extensor branches, directs tension between the dorsal aspect of the digit and the palmar aspect of the metacarpus. In this way, it may facilitate the proximal distribution of impact-related forces and ground reaction forces and the distal distribution of load during weight bearing. The continuity it provides between the structures further suggests that it may decrease the peak tensions applied to the CDET and IL by bearing some of the load and strain that would otherwise be directly applied to them. Hence, perhaps in individuals where this expanse of fascia is thicker or more clearly defined in its fibre orientation, there is greater capacity for weight bearing and force distribution prior to suspensory apparatus breakdown.

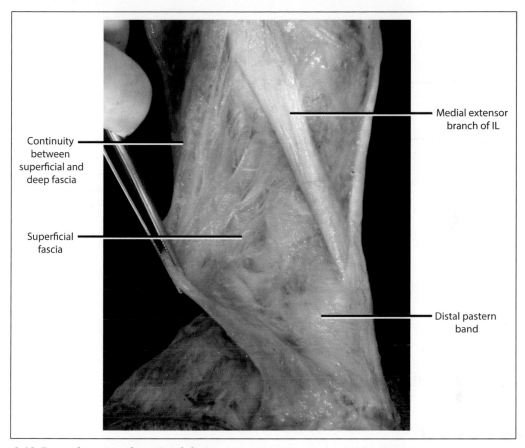

Fig. 3.10 Lateral aspect of proximal digit.

The role of fascia in protecting vessels and nerves

The most common notion surrounding the significance of fascia surrounding vessels and nerves is that it provides a protective sheath to prevent damage that is likely to occur as a result of compression or frictional forces (Benjamin, 2009). However, it is also likely that fascial conduits such as those pictured here act to maintain the position of the vessels and nerves and limit the amount of stretching that may lead to damage or rupture of vessels and nerves, particularly with joint movement. Such a role would be particularly pertinent to the palmar vessels and nerves extending distally over the fetlock joint due to the joint's extreme range of movement.

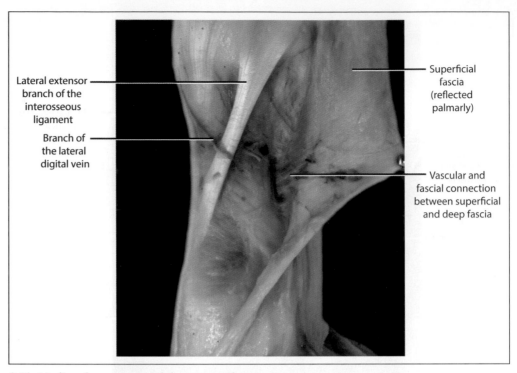

Lateral extensor branch of the interosseous ligament

Branch of the lateral digital vein

Superficial fascia (reflected palmarly)

Vascular and fascial connection between superficial and deep fascia

Fig. 3.11 Mediopalmar aspect of the proximal metacarpus.

Palmar aspect

On the palmar aspect of the Mc3, the superficial fascia is both separate from and intricately connected to, the underlying fascia. A vertical incision made along the mid-length of the SDFT, from the proximal end of the Mc3 to the middle of the annular ligament of the fetlock, reveals that it is easily separable from the underlying deep fascia covering the palmar surface of the SDFT along the entire metacarpus length (**Fig. 3.7**). At the level of the fetlock, the superficial fascia becomes continuous with the deep fascia that covers the flexor tendons in the metacarpal region and together they form a dense connective tissue mass which corresponds in position to the external cornification of skin known as the ergot (**Fig. 3.12**). This fibrous cushion is intimately associated with the skin and has a very firm, inelastic, point of adherence to the annular ligament of the fetlock joint (**Fig. 3.13**). It also serves as the origin for the ligaments of the ergot. A mediopalmar and a lateropalmar ergot ligament exist as clearly defined structures. Each of these have their proximal halves embedded within the superficial fascia and are very closely integrated with the overlying skin (**Fig. 3.14**). Distally, the ligaments of the ergot are continuous with a wide reinforced band of fascia described in more detail in the following.

Over the digital annular ligament, the superficial fascia is loosely adhered (via loose connective tissue). Distally, it then integrates with the perichondrium of the hoof cartilage and the digital cushion.

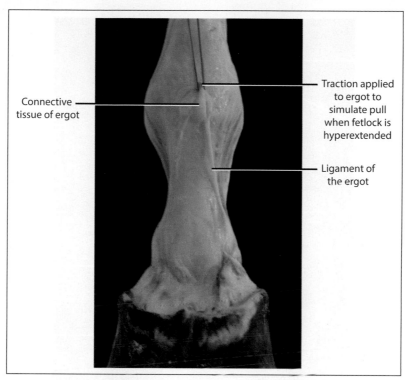

Fig. 3.12 Palmar aspect of the fetlock joint and digit.

The connectivity of the ergot and skin

Proximally, the ergot tissue is continuous with fascia surrounding the flexor tendons, and distally it is continuous with the superficial fascia of the digit (which ultimately blends with the perichondrium of the hoof cartilage). It serves as a junction where fascia of the metacarpus and fascia of the digit unite and further serves as an origin for both superficial and deep fascial layers in these areas. In addition to this, the ergot tissue strongly attaches to the palmar annular ligament of the fetlock joint and thus exists as a central anchored point where fascia and skin of the entire distal limb connect. Traction applied to the ergot tissue in the proximal direction (**Fig. 6.13**) shows how tension is distributed to the distal digital annular ligament, digital cushion and hoof cartilage via the ergot ligaments and their attachment to the distal pastern bands. Hence, the connectivity of the ergot tissue and its derived ligaments suggests three things:

Firstly, that the ergot tissue has a role in the dissipation and absorption of ground reaction forces transmitted up the forelimb by providing an inherent elastic foundation which functions somewhat like a damping pad. In this way, it would act similar to the heel pad of the human foot, which imparts shock absorption properties and helps the heel to resist shear forces (Safran, Garrett, & Seaber, 1988).

Secondly, it suggests that the ergot tissue has a role in maintaining the functional relationship between structures and the connectivity of movement throughout the entire distal forelimb. As described, the ergot tissue serves as a centrally anchored point at which the superficial fascia, deep fascia and skin unite. Each of these layers has expansive connectivity and continuity over the rest of the distal forelimb, which is also likely to extend to the proximal forelimb and the rest of the body. Lastly, the ergot connectivity suggests that the degree of hyperflexion of the fetlock may, to a limited extent, be influenced by the stiffness of the ergot ligaments and skin. Mechanically, the degree of fetlock dorsiflexion is mostly limited by the stiffness of the IL, DDFT and SDFT extending along the palmar aspect of the distal forelimb. The ligaments of the ergot are, in comparison, considerably smaller in both thickness and length, and are therefore likely to have a much smaller mechanical influence on the degree of fetlock dorsiflexion. Instead, their influence is likely to be neurological.

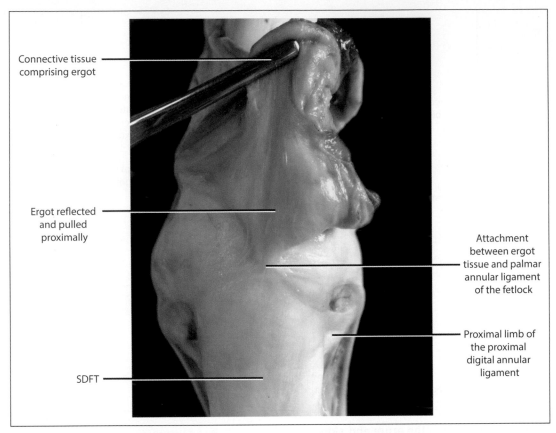

Connective tissue comprising ergot

Ergot reflected and pulled proximally

Attachment between ergot tissue and palmar annular ligament of the fetlock

Proximal limb of the proximal digital annular ligament

SDFT

Fig. 3.13 Palmar aspect of the fetlock joint.

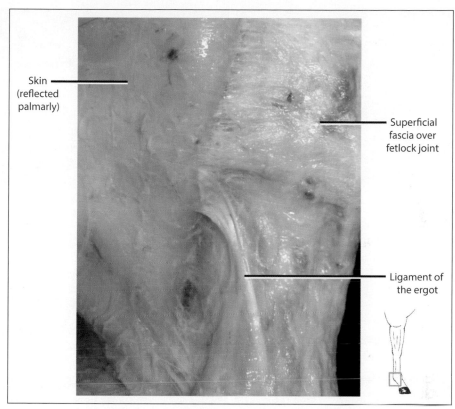

Fig. 3.14 **Connection between the medial ligament of the ergot and the skin on the mediopalmar aspect of the fetlock.**

Ruffini endings

Recent research investigating the role of ligaments in proprioception, suggests that the ligaments of the ergot may serve as proprioceptive structures, which enable communication between connecting structures regarding the position of both the fetlock and pastern joints. The Ruffini endings found in the ergot tissue and ligaments support this hypothesis (**Fig. 3.15**). According to Strong and Elwyn (1948), Ruffini corpuscles characteristically have several nerve fibres, which enter the corpuscle and ramify extensively to record changes in pressure and tension. The presence of these endings in the ergot ligament and tissue strongly suggests a mechanoreceptive function that contributes to positioning of the distal forelimb joints (particularly the fetlock joint).

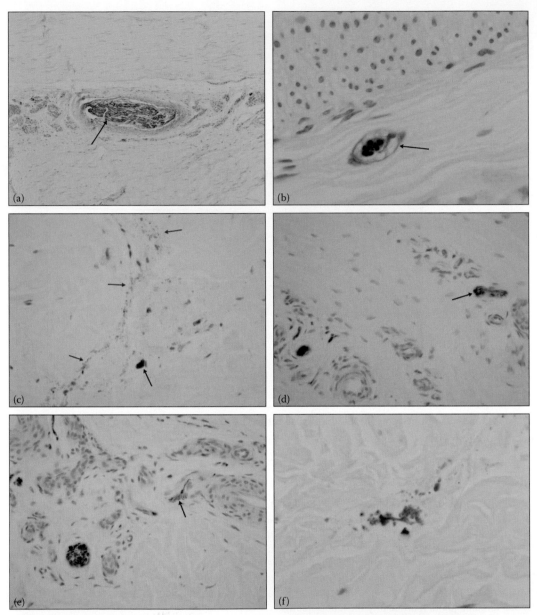

Fig. 3.15 Nerve fibres in the ergot ligament (a–d) and ergot tissue (e–f) detected by S-100 immunohistochemical staining. Arrows in c–f indicate Ruffini endings. Magnification: (a) 10x; (b) 100x; (c) 20x; (d) 100x; (e) 40x; (f) 40x.

DEEP FASCIA

Dorsal, medial and lateral aspects

Deep to the superficial fascia, 1–2 additional fascial layers can be isolated on the dorsal aspect of the Mc3. The most superficial of these – the superficial lamina of deep fascia – is easily identified as it envelops the common and LDETs (**Fig. 3.16**). Similar to the superficial fascia, it appears

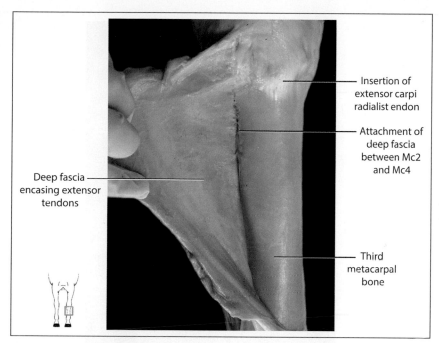

Insertion of extensor carpi radialist endon

Attachment of deep fascia between Mc2 and Mc4

Deep fascia encasing extensor tendons

Third metacarpal bone

Fig. 3.16 Dorsomedial aspect of metacarpus.

grossly to consist of two very closely associated sheets of fascia, which create a clearly defined membrane independent of the overlying superficial fascia.

As alluded to above, this lamina of deep fascia is observed to be continuous with the superficial fascia along the lateral border of the LDET from immediately below the reinforced fascial band connecting the accessory carpal bone to the LDET, to the approximate level of the distal end of Mc4 (**Fig. 3.5**). Dorsomedially, it remains as a distinct layer, which can be isolated from the superficial fascia and the deep lamina of deep fascia situated over the Mc3 periosteal surface (**Fig. 3.16**). On both the medial and lateral aspects, it adheres firmly at the juncture of the Mc3 and the respective splint bone.

Similar to the superficial fascia, the superficial lamina of deep fascia has a largely unspecialised arrangement of fibres over the proximal third of the dorsal Mc3. In the distal two-thirds and situated medial to the CDET, the fibres of this fascia thicken and become oriented in a proximodistal direction, forming a tendon-like band of fascia on approach to the fetlock joint (**Fig. 3.16**). Over the fetlock joint, these vertically arranged fibres are met with oblique fibres which originate and extend from the medial extensor branch of the IL, and together they form a thick fascial connection between the CDET and IL that very closely resembles a ligamentous structure (**Fig. 3.17**). The strength and thickness of these vertical and oblique fibres varies but is generally much greater than that observed over the rest of the deep fascial membrane. Emerging from this expanse of fascia is a strong band, which seems to be of similar, if not greater, thickness and strength than the ergot ligament and which attaches to the periosteal surface of the proximal extremity of the proximal phalanx (**Figs. 3.18** and **3.19**).

A similar oblique orientation of fibres is observed extending from the lateral IL extensor branch on the lateral aspect of the fetlock. These fibres are of similar thickness to those apparent on the medial aspect and appear macroscopically to be continuous over the dorsolateral aspect of the fetlock joint with the distal extremity of the LDET (**Fig. 3.20**).

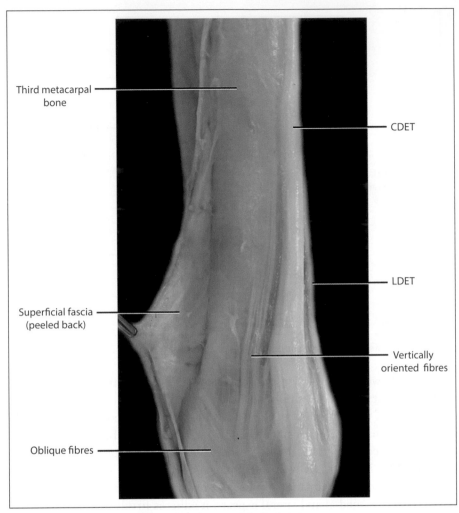

Third metacarpal bone

CDET

LDET

Superficial fascia (peeled back)

Vertically oriented fibres

Oblique fibres

Fig. 3.17 **Dorsomedial aspect of the metacarpus and fetlock joint.**

Associated with the fascia and tendons of the dorsal aspect of the fetlock are 2–3 bursae. On the medial side, a subfascial bursa is observed in three specimens, approximately 1.0 cm in diameter (**Figs. 3.18** and **3.21**). Deep to the combined common and LDETs a subtendinous bursa is present (**Figs. 3.22** and **3.23**); as is a small subtendinous bursa situated deep to the LDET (**Fig. 3.24**).

Distal to the fetlock, the deep fascia is inseparable from the distal extensions of the medial and lateral IL extensor branches. In the region of the middle phalanx, it forms a reinforced band on the medial and lateral aspects, which are connected to the CDET and IL extensor branches (**Fig. 3.25**). These bands (distal pastern bands) are continuous with the ligaments of the ergot on each side and have attachments to the hoof cartilage and the digital cushion on the palmar aspect (**Figs. 3.26** and **3.27**).

The deep lamina of deep fascia is exceptionally thin and is not easily separable from the dorsal periosteal surface of the Mc3. On gross observation, it has a highly irregular arrangement of collagen fibres. Proximally, it blends with the insertion of the extensor carpi radialis tendon as well as the carpal fascia, which wraps around the palmar aspect of the Mc3.

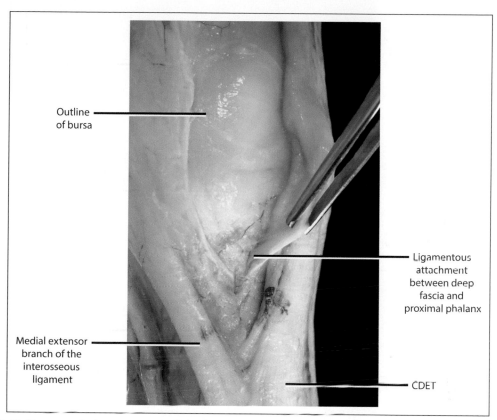

Outline of bursa

Ligamentous attachment between deep fascia and proximal phalanx

Medial extensor branch of the interosseous ligament

CDET

Fig. 3.18 Dorsomedial aspect of the fetlock joint.

Proprioception in the distal forelimb

The highly specialised and consistent organisation of fascia over the dorsolateral and dorsomedial aspects of the fetlock joint may indicate that it has proprioceptive support functions which help maintain the joint range of motion within a physiological range. Studies in humans and cats have revealed proprioceptive nerve endings within fascia and ligaments surrounding highly mobile joints. The presence of such nerve endings in soft connective tissue structures surrounding joints suggests that joints have an intrinsic ability to maintain their movement within a range where breakdown is less likely to occur. Being a highly mobile diarthrodial joint, it is possible that the expanse of fascia between the extensors and the IL over the dorsomedial and dorsolateral aspects of the fetlock joint contain proprioceptive nerve endings that are important in the overall arthrokinetics of the fetlock joint. Furthermore, there is an emerging area of research investigating the role of mechanical connections across and between joints in providing inherent stability to joints during rapid locomotion. Studies investigating this suggest that mechanical fascial connections may respond more rapidly to impact-related perturbations than neural reflex mechanisms. Hence, the fascial expansions over the fetlock joint may contribute to stability of the distal limb at fast speeds by providing mechanical linkages through which tension can be easily distributed.

Distally it becomes involved with the superficial lamina of deep fascia to form the subtendinous bursa over the fetlock joint and the fetlock joint capsule. It also blends with the medial and lateral collateral ligaments of the fetlock towards the distal end of the Mc3. Similar to the superficial fascia and superficial lamina of deep fascia, the deep lamina merges with fascia surrounding the palmar vessels and nerves in the distal third of the metacarpus.

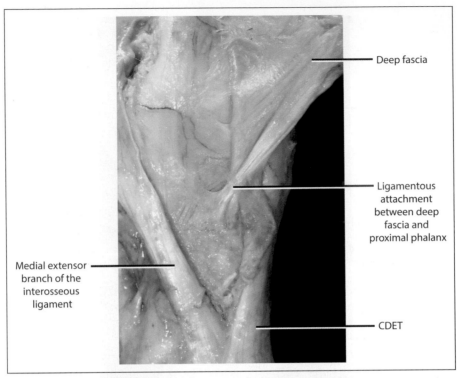

Fig. 3.19 Connectivity of the deep fascia over the dorsomedial aspect of the fetlock joint.

Deep fascia

Ligamentous attachment between deep fascia and proximal phalanx

Medial extensor branch of the interosseous ligament

CDET

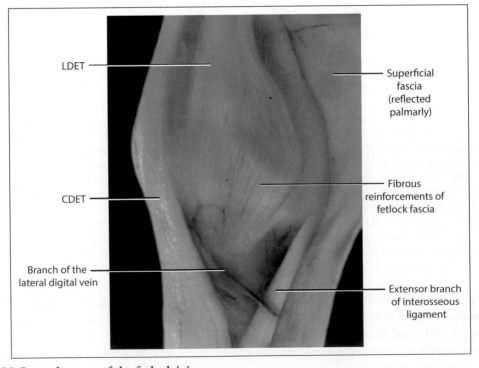

Fig. 3.20 Lateral aspect of the fetlock joint.

LDET

Superficial fascia (reflected palmarly)

Fibrous reinforcements of fetlock fascia

CDET

Branch of the lateral digital vein

Extensor branch of interosseous ligament

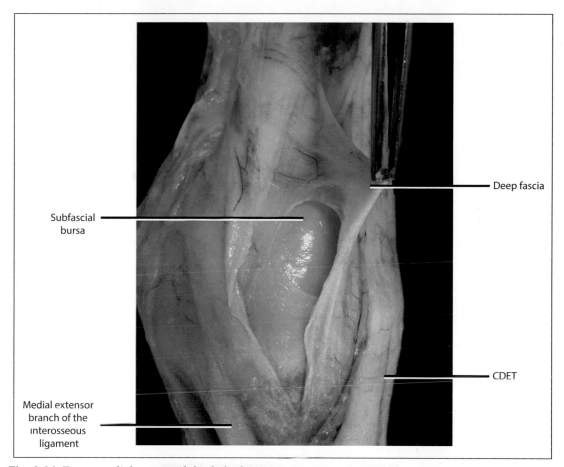

Deep fascia

Subfascial
bursa

CDET

Medial extensor
branch of the
interosseous
ligament

Fig. 3.21 Dorsomedial aspect of the fetlock joint.

Bursae

The deep fascia is involved in forming several bursae around the fetlock joint. Most of these have already been described in the literature. However, an exception to this is the subfascial bursae on the dorsomedial aspect of the fetlock joint. This bursa was inconsistently observed among specimens and therefore it is possible that it is only present in exceptionally rare occasions or that it develops in response to particular mechanical loads.

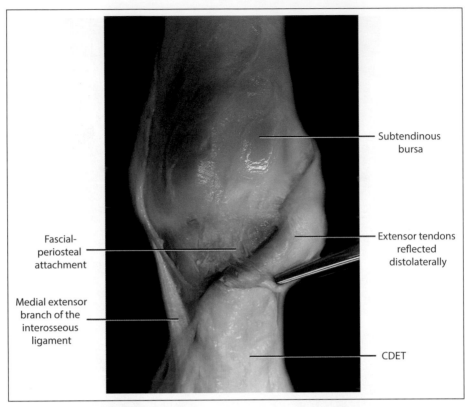

Subtendinous bursa

Extensor tendons reflected distolaterally

Fascial-periosteal attachment

Medial extensor branch of the interosseous ligament

CDET

Fig. 3.22 **Dorsal aspect of the fetlock joint.**

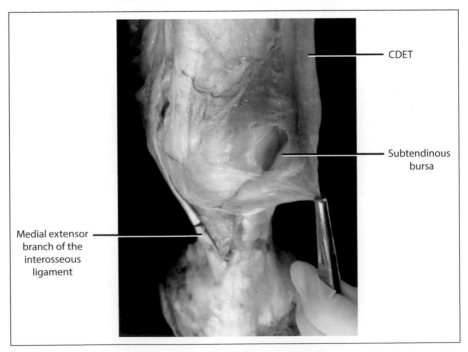

CDET

Subtendinous bursa

Medial extensor branch of the interosseous ligament

Fig. 3.23 **Dorsomedial aspect of the fetlock joint viewed proximally.**

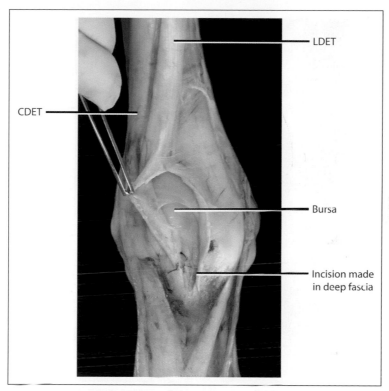

Fig. 3.24 Dorsolateral aspect of the fetlock joint.

Distal pastern bands

The reinforced fascial bands on the medial and lateral aspects of the middle phalanx are likely to have a role in load distribution. To our knowledge, the existence of these bands has only been acknowledged once in the existing literature in a series of detailed sketches by Schmaltz (1911). In his work, these fascial bands are referred to as *untere dorsale fesselbinde* (distal dorsal pastern bands) and are continuous dorsally with the medial and lateral edges of the CDET, and palmarly with the distal digital annular ligament, hoof cartilage, and digital cushion (**Fig. 6.36**). The digital cushion itself is thought to absorb concussive forces associated with ground impact. Through the distal pastern band, a small magnitude of these forces may be redirected to the CDET and the IL to ensure a more even distribution of tensional forces.

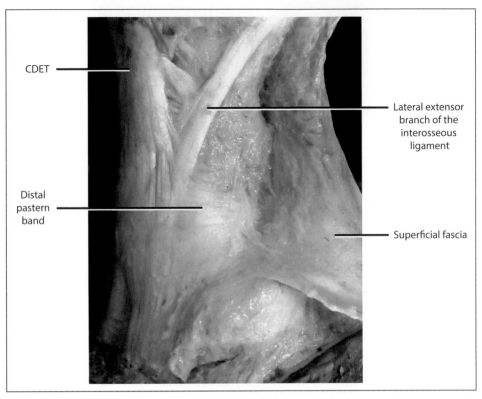

Fig. 3.25 Dorsolateral aspect of the equine proximal digit.

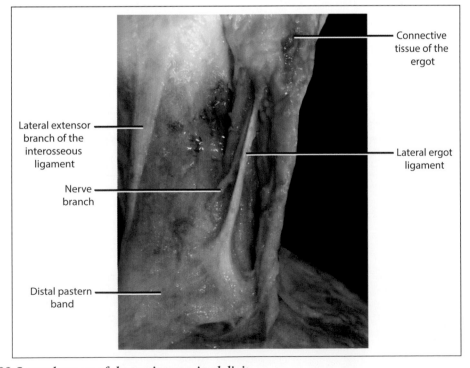

Fig. 3.26 Lateral aspect of the equine proximal digit.

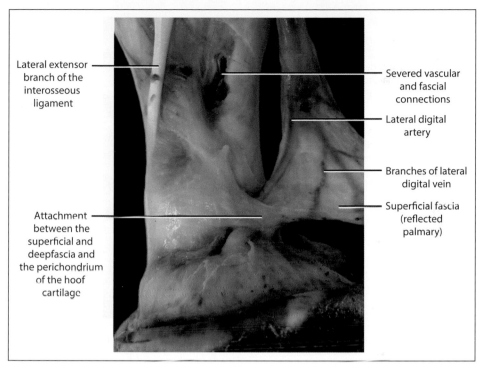

Lateral extensor branch of the interosseous ligament

Severed vascular and fascial connections

Lateral digital artery

Branches of lateral digital vein

Superficial fascia (reflected palmary)

Attachment between the superficial and deepfascia and the perichondrium of the hoof cartilage

Fig. 3.27 Lateral aspect of the equine proximal digit. Superficial fascia has been reflected palmarly.

Palmar aspect

A longitudinal incision made along the palmar length of the SDFT, reveals the deep fascia surrounding the flexor tendons to be intricately organised along the length of the Mc3. Proximally and deep to the superficial lamina already described, a thick, strong sheet passes from Mc2 to Mc4 (**Fig. 3.28**). This sheet is continuous over the surface of the interosseous ligament (**Fig. 3.29**) and thus maintains their position along the proximal palmar aspect of Mc3 (**Fig. 3.28**). When followed

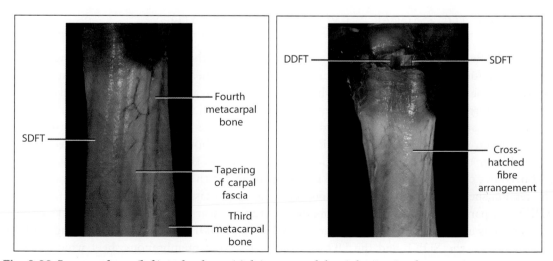

SDFT

Fourth metacarpal bone

Tapering of carpal fascia

Third metacarpal bone

DDFT

SDFT

Cross-hatched fibre arrangement

Fig. 3.28 Lateropalmar (left) and palmar (right) aspect of the right proximal metacarpus.

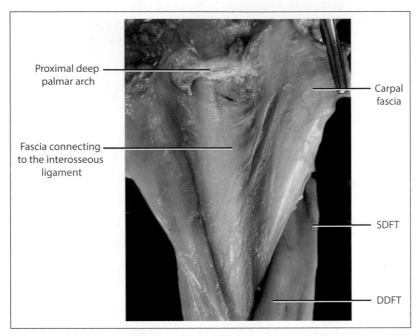

Proximal deep palmar arch

Carpal fascia

Fascia connecting to the interosseous ligament

SDFT

DDFT

Fig. 3.29 **Palmar aspect of the metacarpus with the flexor tendons removed.**

proximally, it is a clear distal extension of the carpal fascia, which has reinforced fibres forming the flexor retinaculum of the carpal joint. At the proximal end of the Mc3, this extension of the carpal fascia has a cross-hatched arrangement of fibres oriented distolaterally and distomedially, and which tapers along the axial surfaces of the Mc2 and the Mc4 (**Fig. 3.28**). Between these tapered points of reinforced fascia, the fascia continues distally, thinning along the way. At the fetlock joint, it merges with the superficial fascia and the dense connective tissue mass comprising the ergot. This connective tissue has a strong, inelastic attachment to the palmar annular ligament of the fetlock joint and serves as a prominent point of juncture for the superficial and deep fascia expanding over the entire distal forelimb (**Fig. 3.13**).

FASCIA OF THE CARPAL FLEXOR TENDON SHEATH

Around the flexor tendons in the proximal third of the Mc3, there is an intricate arrangement of fascia which forms the distal part of the carpal flexor tendon sheath (**Fig. 3.30**). The distal boundary of this sheath occurs at the point where the accessory ligament of the DDFT (distal check ligament) merges with the DDFT (around or slightly proximal to the mid-metacarpus). Proximal to this point of merging, the parietal and visceral layers of the sheath can be distinguished. The parietal layer, which lies deep to the thick carpal fascia as shown in **Fig. 3.30**, connects to the visceral layer through the medial palmar artery. It encircles the flexor tendons until it reaches and becomes continuous with the distal check ligament. In this way, it forms the dorsal wall of the tendon sheath and becomes continuous with the carpal fascia. On the palmar surface of the SDFT, the parietal layer thins distally and encases the metacarpal communicating nerve branch. It remains as an enveloping sheet around the SDFT and DDFT along the entire length of the Mc3. Between the SDFT and the DDFT, it gives rise to a membranous sheet which extends between the SDFT and DDFT immediately distal to the point of juncture between the DDFT

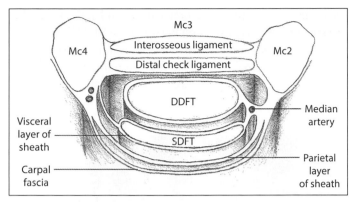

Fig. 3.30 **Sketch of the fascial layers around metacarpus.**

and the distal check ligament. Medial and lateral to the flexor tendons in the distal third of the Mc3, it joins with the fascial hiatus which surrounds the palmar vessels and nerves. This fascia invests between the deep flexor tendon and the IL to encase the nerves of the distal palmar arch at the bifurcation point of the IL (**Fig. 3.31**).

The visceral layer of the carpal tendon sheath surrounds the SDFT and DDFT in the region of the proximal third of the Mc3. The mesotendon formed between the two flexor tendons is via the fascia surrounding the medial palmar artery and nerve. Its position of attachment to the DDFT varies. Often, it can be observed on its medial side or mediopalmar side, but occasionally it can be observed attaching along the midline of the tendon. It remains inseparable from the epitenon

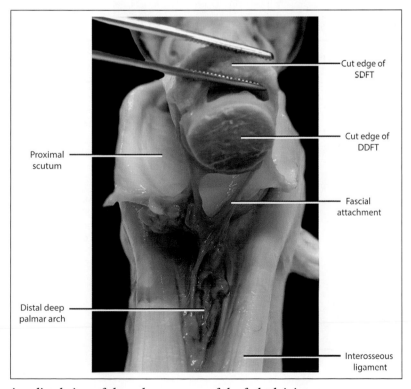

Fig. 3.31 **Proximodistal view of the palmar aspect of the fetlock joint.**

of the flexor tendons along the length of the metacarpus and fetlock. In the distal third of the metacarpus, it forms a strong fibrous connection between the SDFT and the DDFT which marks the proximal boundary of the sesamoidean part of the digital flexor tendon sheath (**Fig. 3.32**). The distal boundary of the metacarpal part of the flexor tendon sheath is formed by the merging of the annular ligament to the SDFT (**Fig. 3.33**).

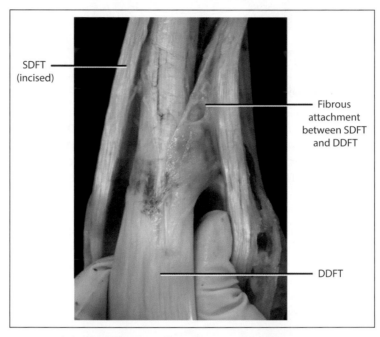

SDFT (incised)

Fibrous attachment between SDFT and DDFT

DDFT

Fig. 3.32 Palmar aspect of the distal metacarpus.

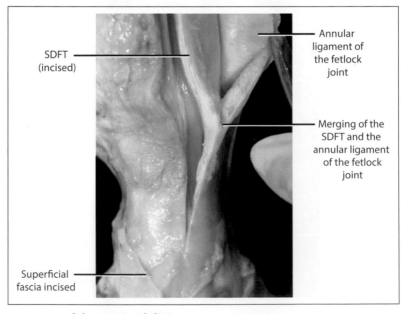

SDFT (incised)

Annular ligament of the fetlock joint

Merging of the SDFT and the annular ligament of the fetlock joint

Superficial fascia incised

Fig. 3.33 Palmar aspect of the proximal digit.

At the approximate distal end of the proximal phalanx, a membranous sheet spans across the two extensions of the SDFT, deep to the DDFT. Small tendon-like connections termed *vincula tendinea* emerge from this membranous sheet and connect the DDFT to both the SDFT and the straight sesamoidean ligament (**Figs. 3.34** and **3.35**).

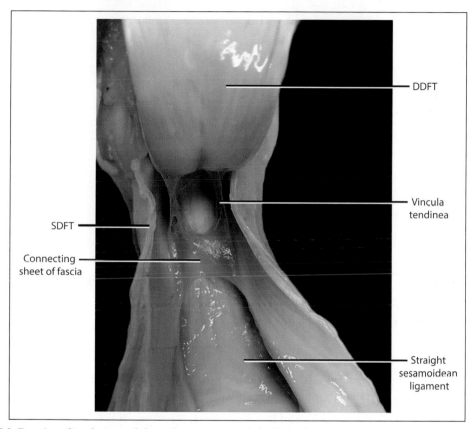

Fig. 3.34 **Proximodistal view of the palmar aspect of the fetlock joint.**

Vincula tendinea

These pictured connections, termed *vincula tendinea*, are common in the human hand and are important in the vascular supply of the superficial and deep digital flexor tendons (Stewart et al., 2007). Furthermore, they have been found to facilitate digital flexion after distal tendon transection in cadaveric human hands, allowing tendons to act indirectly across the interphalangeal joints (Stewart et al., 2007). Vincula tendinea in the equine digit have not been described in detail but are thought to act as a means of uniting parietal and visceral layers of the tendon sheath, with their main function being to carry vessels and nerves. The vincula tendinea pictured above most likely support a vascular supply to the straight sesamoidean ligament, the DDFT and the SDFT. The biomechanical role of these thin fibrous connections in flexion and extension of the joint is difficult to assess, but is unlikely to be as remarkable as that in the human hand due to differences in digit use and the highly specialised design of the equine digit.

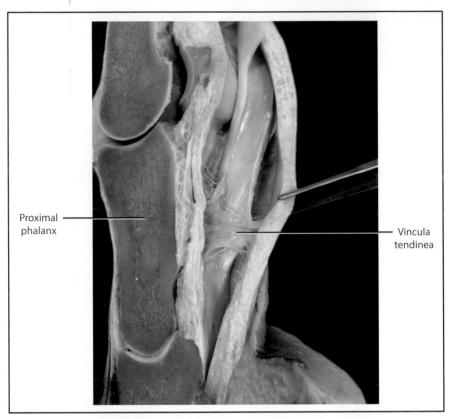

Proximal phalanx

Vincula tendinea

Fig. 3.35 **Mid-sagittal section of the equine proximal digit.**

REFERENCES

Benjamin, M. (2009). The fascia of the limbs and back- a review. *Journal of Anatomy, 214,* 1–18.

Bowsher, C., Steer, M., & Tobin, A. (2008). *Plant Biochemistry.* New York, NY: Garland Science, Taylor & Francis Group.

Guimberteau, J., Delage, J., & Wong, J. (2010). The role and mechanical behaviour of the connective tissue in tendon sliding. *Chirurgie de la main, 29,* 155–166.

Safran, M., Garrett, W. J., & Seaber, A. (1988). The role of warm-up in muscular injury prevention. *American Journal of Sports Medicine, 16*(2), 123–129.

Smith, H. (1977). *The Molecular Biology of Plant Cells* (Vol. 14). Berkeley: University of California Press.

Stecco, C. (2015). *Functional Atlas of the Human Fascial System.* Edinburgh: Elsevier.

BIBLIOGRAPHY

Back, W., Schamhardt, H., Savelberg, H., van den Bogert, A., Bruin, G., Hartman, W., & Barneveld, A. (1995). How the horse moves: 1. Significance of graphical representations of equine forelimb kinematics. *Equine Veterinary Journal, 27*(1), 31–38.

Balch, O., Butler, D., White, K., & Metcalf, S. (1995). Hoof balance and lameness: Improper toe length, hoof angle, and mediolateral balance. *The Compendium on Continuing Education for the Practicing Veterinarian, 17*(10), 1275–1278.

Barone, R. (2010). *Arthrologie et Myologie* (4th ed., Vol. 2). Paris: Éditions Vigot.

Boyde, A., & Roberts, T. (1953). Proprioceptive discharges from stretch-receptors in the knee-joint of the cat. *Journal of Physiology, 122*, 38–58.

Clayton, H., Lanovaz, J., Schamhardt, H., Willemen, M., & Colborne, G. (1998). Net joint moments and powers in the equine forelimb during the stance phase of the trot. *Equine Veterinary Journal, 30*(5), 384–389.

Dimery, N., Alexander, R., & Ker, R. (1986). Elastic extension of leg tendons in the locomotion of horses *(Equus caballus)*. *Journal of Zoology, 210*(1), 415–425.

Dyce, K., Sack, W., & Wensing, C. (2002). *Textbook of Veterinary Anatomy* (3rd ed.). Philadelphia, PA: W.B. Saunders.

Eng, J., Winter, D., & Patla, A. (1996). Intralimb dynamics simplify recative control strategies during locomotion. *Journal of Biomechanics, 30*(6), 581–588.

Herring, L., Thompson, K., & Jarret, S. (1992). Defining normal 3-dimensional kinematics of the lower forelimb in horses. *Equine Veterinary Science, 12*(3), 172–176.

Holmström, M., & Philipsson, J. (1993). Relationships between conformation, performance and health in 4 year old Swedish warmblood riding horses. *Livestock Production Science, 33*(3–4), 293–312. doi:10.1016/0301-6226(93)90009-7

Jeffcott, L., Rossdale, P., Freestone, J., Frank, C., & Towers-Clark, P. (1982). An assessment of wastage in Thoroughbred racing from conception to 4 years of age. *Equine Veterinary Journal, 14*(3), 185–198.

Jerosch, J., & Prymka, M. (1996). Proprioception and joint stability. *Knee Surgery, Sports Traumatology, Arthroscopy, 4*, 171–179.

König, H., Liebich, H., & Bragulla, H. (2007). *Veterinary Anatomy of Domestic Mammals: Textbook and Colour Atlas*. Stuttgart: Schattauer.

Langevin, H. (2006). Connective tissue: A body-wide signaling network? *Medical Hypotheses, 66*, 1074–1077.

Marcus, A., & Kuchera, M. (2004). *Foundations for Integrative Musculoskeletal Medicine: An East-West Approach*. Berkeley, CA: North Atlantic Books.

McIlwraith, C., Frisbie, D., Kawcak, C., & van Weeren, P. (1996). *Joint Disease in the Horse* (2nd ed.). St. Louis, MO: Elsevier.

Michelson, J., & Hutchins, C. (1995). Mechanoreceptors in human ankle ligaments. *Journal of Bone and Joint Surgery, 77-B*(2), 219–224.

Minetti, A., Ardigo, L., Reinach, E., & Saibene, F. (1999). The relationship between mechanical work and energy expenditure of locomotion in horses. *Journal of Experimental Biology, 202*, 2329–2338.

Moritz, C., & Farley, C. (2004). Passive dynamics change leg mechanics for an unexpected surface during human hopping. *Journal of Applied Physiology, 97*, 1313–1322.

Myers, T. (1997). The 'anatomy trains'. *Journal of Bodywork and Movement Therapies, 1*(2), 91–101.

Nickel, R., Schummer, A., Seiferle, E., Wilkens, H., Wille, K.-H., & Frewein, J. (1986). *The Anatomy of the Domestic Mammals* (Vol. 1). Berlin: Verlag Paul Parey.

Oteh, U. (2008). *Mechanics of Fluids*. Bloomington, IN: AuthorHouse.

Ottoway, C., & Worden, A. (1940). Bursae and tendon sheaths of the horse. *Veterinary Records, 52*(26), 477–483.

Patla, A., & Prentice, S. (1995). The role of active forces and intersegmental dynamics in the control of limb trajectory over obstacles during locomotion in humans. *Experimental Brain Research, 106*, 499–504.

Perkins, N., Reid, S., & Morris, R. (2004). Profiling the New Zealand Thoroughbred racing industry. 2. Conditions interfering with training and racing. *New Zealand Veterinary Journal, 53*(1), 69–76.

Schleip, R., Klingler, W., & Lehmann-Horn, F. (2005). Active fascial contractility: Fascia may be able to contract in a smooth muscle-like manner and thereby influence musculoskeletal dynamics. *Medical Hypotheses, 65*(2), 273–277.

Schmaltz, R. (1911). *Atlas der Anatomie des Pferdes: Topographische Myologie* (Vol. 2). Berlin: Verlagsbuchhandlung von Richard Schoetz.

Schultz, R., Miller, D., Kerr, C., & Micheli, L. (1984). Mechanoreceptors in human cruciate ligaments. *Journal of Bone and Joint Surgery, 66*(7), 1072–1076.

Sisson, S., & Grossman, J. (1938). *The Anatomy of the Domestic Animals* (3rd ed.). Philadelphia, PA: W.B. Saunders.

Stecco, C., Macchi, V., Porzionato, A., Morra, A., Parenti, A., Stecco, A., ... De Caro, R. (2010). The ankle retinacula: Morphological evidence of the proprioceptive role of the fascial system. *Cells Tissues Organs, 192*, 200–210.

Stephens, P., Nunamaker, D., & Butterweck, D. (1989). Application of a Hall-effect transducer for measurement of tendon strains in horses. *American Journal of Veterinary Research, 50*(7), 1089–1095.

Stewart, D. A., Smitham, P. J., Gianoutsos, M. P., & Walsh, W. R. (2007). Biomechanical influence of the vincula tendinum on digital motion after isolated flexor tendon injury: a cadaveric study. *Journal of Hand Surgery, 32*(8), 1190–1194.

Strong, O., & Elwyn, A. (1948). Peripheral Terminations of afferent nerve fibres. In M. Baltimore (Ed.), *Human Neuroanatomy* (2nd ed.), pp. 68–80. United States: Williams and Wilkins.

Williams, R., Harkins, L., Hammond, C., & Wood, J. (2001). Racehorse injuries, clinical problems and fatalities recorded on British racecourses from flat racing and National Hunt racing during 1996, 1997 and 1998. *Equine Veterinary Journal, 33*(5), 478–486.

Wilson, A., McGuigan, M., Su, A., & van den Bogert, A. (2001). Horses damp the spring in their step. *Nature, 414*, 895–899.

Wilson, A., Watson, J., & Lichtwark, G. (2003). Biomechanics: A catapult action for rapid limb protraction. *Nature, 421*(6918), 35–36.

CHAPTER 4

FASCIA OF THE EQUINE ANTEBRACHIUM

INTRODUCTION

Generally, much of the research directed at understanding the biomechanical importance of the antebrachium has focused on its musculoskeletal anatomy. The skeletal anatomy in particular effectively contributes to the overall shock-absorbing and load-bearing capacity of the forelimb, as well as adding (a variable amount) to the overall forward impulse (Badoux, 1974). This is made possible by the fixed positioning of the radius and ulna, which enables full load to be carried by the radius in the support phase, rather than being transmitted to the humeral trochlea and absorbed through the radioulnar interosseous membrane as occurs in man. In addition to this, the relative immobility of the radius and ulna maintains a consistent alignment with the mechanical line of the distal forelimb and therefore further reduces twisting forces which may otherwise predispose the antebrachium to overuse and strain injury (Badoux, 1974).

In relation to the musculature of the antebrachium, several studies have investigated the architecture and histological properties of individual muscles or functional groups of muscles such as the superficial and deep digital flexors (Brown, Pandy, Buford, Kawcak, & McIlwraith, 2003; Butcher et al., 2009; Hermanson & Cobb, 1992; Zarucco, Taylor, & Stover, 2004). These studies are limited in that they functionally isolate these muscles and only consider their effects in terms of their direct tendinous extensions and attachments. Hence, they fail to consider the role of connecting fascial tissues in mediating the transmission of force between muscles or even between muscles and bones.

Unfortunately, the descriptive details provided for fascial characteristics of the antebrachium have been inconsistent among authors and therefore deducing the functional significance of the antebrachial fascia has been difficult. The number of fascial compartments illustrated or described in the antebrachium is one such example of this inconsistency; another is in the variable identification of superficial and deep fascial layers.

Furthermore, and perhaps more importantly from a functional perspective, there has been no attempt to discuss the possible paths of force and tension distribution and how the fascial organisation and connectivity may mechanically coordinate the function of several discrete elements. This is an aspect of the functional antebrachial anatomy which is essential to elucidate, in order to thoroughly understand the overall biomechanics of the limb.

In consideration of the entire forelimb, the antebrachium exists as the intermediate segment between the distal forelimb and the shoulder girdle and brachium. Hence, the transmission of forces throughout the fascia of the antebrachium is likely to facilitate coordination of the proximal and distal limb segments and to contribute to the overall stability of the limb.

Investigation into the fascial connectivity therefore has the potential to further the current understanding of forelimb biomechanics and postural control.

ANTEBRACHIAL FASCIA: SUMMARY

Both superficial and deep fascial layers are present in the equine antebrachium. The superficial fascia encases the whole antebrachium in a stocking-like manner, with particular areas of notable attachment described in the following. Proximally, it is continuous with the superficial fascia of the brachium (**Figs. 4.1–4.3**), whilst distally it is continuous with the superficial fascia of the metacarpus (**Fig. 4.4**). It can generally be relatively easily separated from the overlying skin due to the delicate nature of the loose connective tissue in between the two layers. An example of this is given in **Fig. 4.5**. In contrast, more fibrous connectivity exists between the skin and superficial fascia over the olecranon process of the ulna (**Fig. 4.6**).

The deep fascia can be isolated as two to three separate laminae along different aspects of the antebrachium and generally invests between muscles to create isolated muscular compartments. These are described in detail in the following.

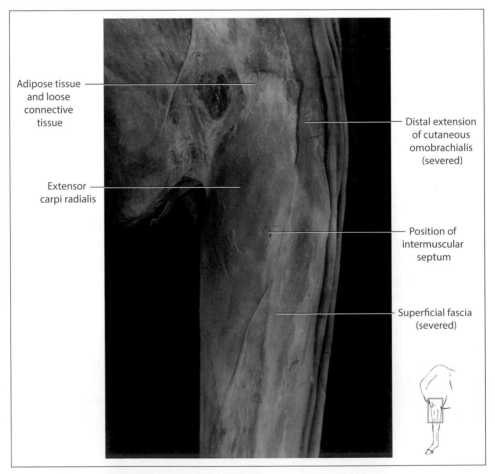

Fig. 4.1 Dorsolateral aspect of the left antebrachium.

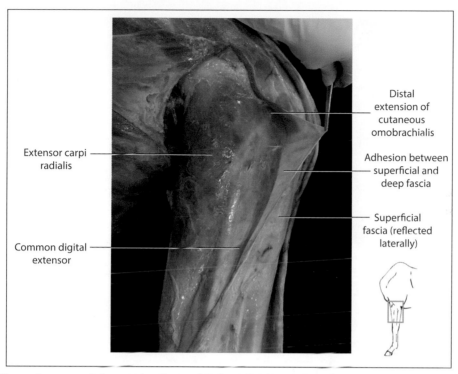

Distal extension of cutaneous omobrachialis

Adhesion between superficial and deep fascia

Superficial fascia (reflected laterally)

Extensor carpi radialis

Common digital extensor

Fig. 4.2 Lateral aspect of the proximal two-thirds of the left antebrachium.

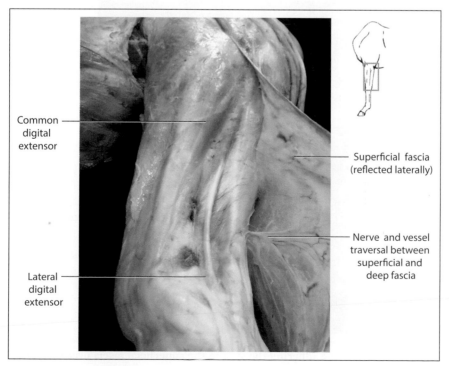

Common digital extensor

Lateral digital extensor

Superficial fascia (reflected laterally)

Nerve and vessel traversal between superficial and deep fascia

Fig. 4.3 Dorsolateral aspect of the left carpus and antebrachium.

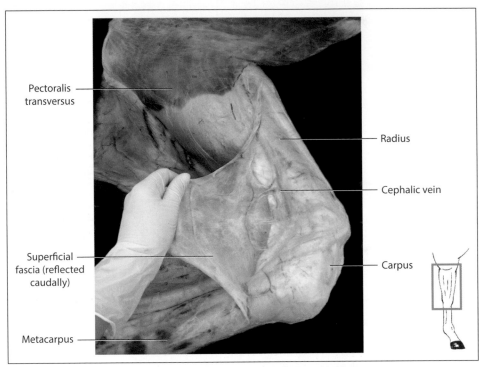

Fig. 4.4 Medial aspect of left antebrachium and proximal half of the metacarpus.

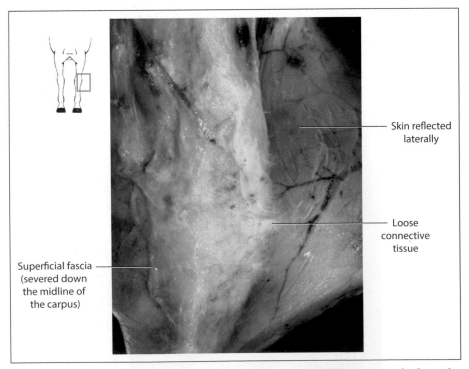

Fig. 4.5 Loose connective tissue adhering the skin to the superficial fascia over the lateral aspect of the left carpus.

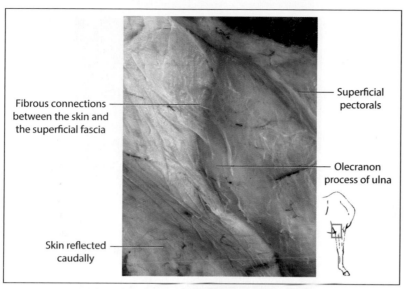

Fig. 4.6 Lateral aspect of the right elbow joint showing the fibrous connectivity between the superficial fascia and the overlying skin.

SUPERFICIAL FASCIA

Medial aspect

The superficial fascia over the medial aspect of the antebrachium covers the medial surface of the radius as well as the deep fascia encasing the flexor carpi radialis (FCR) muscle. Proximally, at a point slightly distal to the cubital joint, it provides insertion for the pectoralis transversus muscle (with which it is continuous) and subsequently it continues as the superficial fascia of the brachium (**Figs. 4.7** and **4.8**). Within the distal region of the pectoralis transversus muscle,

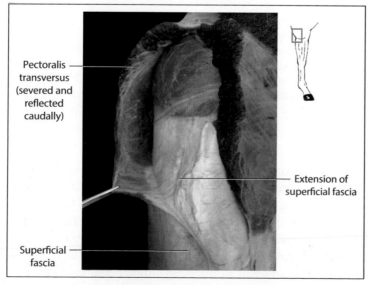

Fig. 4.7 Medial aspect of proximal antebrachium (left forelimb). Superficial fascia (and the pectoralis transversus) have been transected in order to show the relationship with tensor fascia antebrachii.

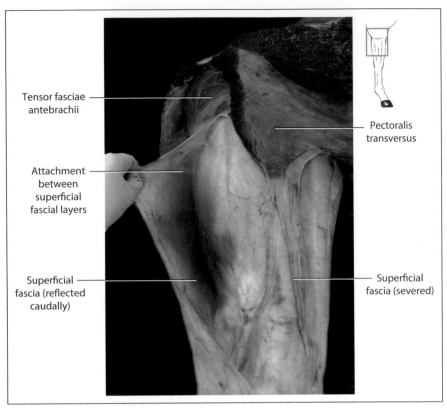

Tensor fasciae antebrachii

Attachment between superficial fascial layers

Superficial fascia (reflected caudally)

Pectoralis transversus

Superficial fascia (severed)

Fig. 4.8 Medial aspect of proximal antebrachium showing connectivity between the superficial and deep fascial layers distal to the elbow joint (left forelimb).

Tensor fasciae antebrachii

The TFA finds insertion in the superficial fascia slightly proximal to the pectoralis transversus and also strongly attaches on its deep surface to the underlying deep antebrachial fascia. The TFA arises from the caudal border of the scapula by means of a broad aponeurosis and also by means of a tendinous sheet from the terminal tendon of the latissimus dorsi.

Taking these connections into account, tensional forces distributing through the TFA or being initiated through its contractility in a live animal can be directed to, from, or between the antebrachium, brachium, shoulder girdle and even the trunk through its fascial connectivity.

---

the superficial fascia becomes complicated in its attachment to the underlying deep antebrachial fascia. **Fig. 4.9** illustrates a consistent, single resilient attachment connecting the underside of the pectoralis transversus to the underlying fascial layer. Adding to the complexity of this fascial arrangement, a second fascial sheet is continuous with the tensor fascia antebrachii (TFA) and biceps brachii proximally (**Figs. 4.7, 4.8** and **4.10**). This secondary layer blends with the fascia extending from the pectoralis transversus distally between the proximal and middle thirds of the antebrachium and is strongly attached to the deep antebrachial fascia on the underside of the TFA. In this way, there is minimal room for movement between the fascial planes over the medial aspect of the proximal antebrachium (**Figs. 4.11** and **4.12**).

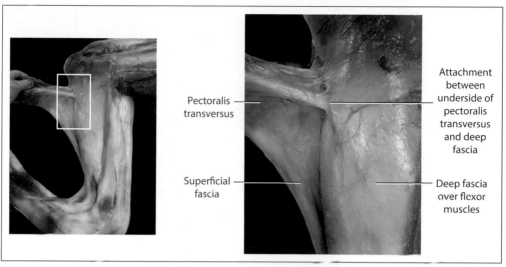

Fig. 4.9 Attachment between the superficial fascia on the underside of the pectoralis transversus muscle and the deep fascia over the caudomedial aspect of the left proximal antebrachium.

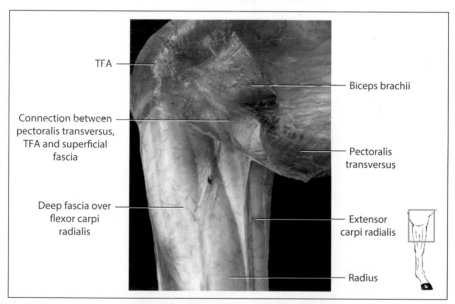

Fig. 4.10 Fascial connectivity over the cranial and medial aspects of the left proximal antebrachium.

As it courses distally from the pectoralis transversus and TFA, the superficial fascia thins slightly but can still be separated from the deep fascia over the medial aspect of the distal antebrachium and carpus. Over the carpal region in particular, the connection between the superficial and deep fascial layers is neither particularly strong nor robust; however, communication between the layers is maintained via small traversing nerve branches and vessels as shown in **Figs. 4.13** and **4.14**.

The accessory branch of the cephalic vein, which terminates immediately proximal to, or in the proximal region of, the carpus can be found encased within the superficial fascia over the medial surface of the radius caudal to the extensor carpi radialis (ECR). Its main branch is situated caudal

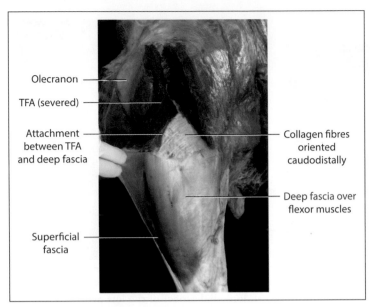

Fig. 4.11 Caudomedial aspect of the left antebrachium with the pectoralis transversus removed.

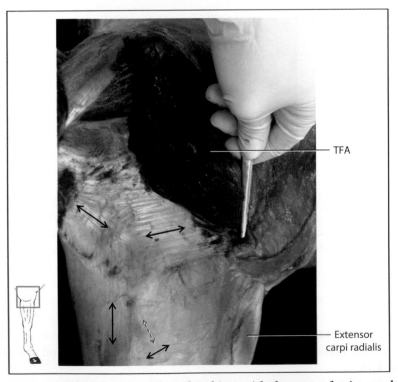

Fig. 4.12 Medial aspect of the left proximal antebrachium with the tensor fasciae antebrachii severed and the caudal half removed. Arrows show the alignment of collagen fibres in the antebrachial fascia (dotted grey arrow shows fibre orientation in underlying fascial layer).

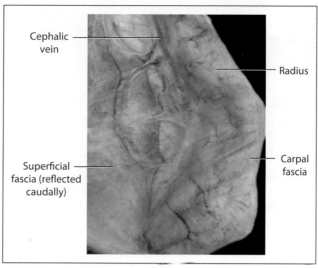

Cephalic vein

Radius

Superficial fascia (reflected caudally)

Carpal fascia

Fig. 4.13 **Medial aspect of the left carpus.**

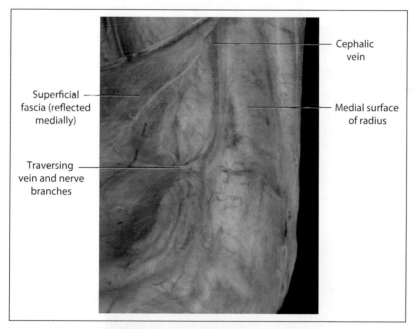

Cephalic vein

Superficial fascia (reflected medially)

Medial surface of radius

Traversing vein and nerve branches

Fig. 4.14 **Medial aspect of the left distal antebrachium and carpus.**

to the accessory branch and is, in contrast, encased within the deep fascia. It only fuses with the superficial fascia in the most proximal region of the forearm as shown in **Fig. 4.15**. A second point of connection between the superficial and deep fascia occurs in the distal third of the antebrachium, where a branch of the cephalic vein passes between layers (**Fig. 4.14**).

The orientation of collagen fibres comprising the superficial fascia over the medial aspect is mostly irregular. However, immediately caudal to the accessory branch of the cephalic vein, a distinct parallel arrangement of fibres is present from the distal insertion of the pectoralis transversus muscle, to the distal third of the radius (**Fig. 4.16**). These fibres are directed craniodistally

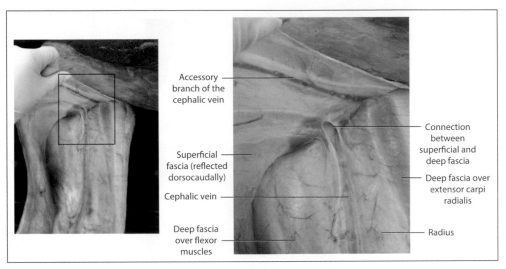

Fig. 4.15 Medial aspect of the proximal antebrachium. Magnified image shows the relationship between the superficial and deep fascial layers of the antebrachium.

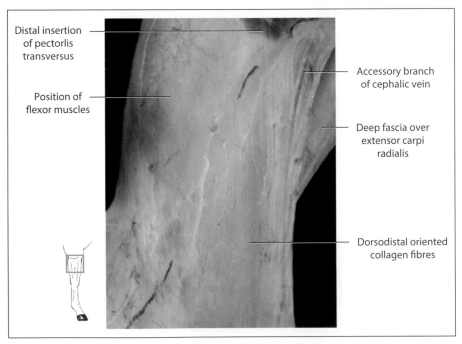

Fig. 4.16 Superficial fascia over the caudomedial aspect of the left proximal antebrachium.

and demonstrate a strong resistance to stretch in response to traction applied distally. They also provide the thickest and strongest expanse of superficial fascia over the entire antebrachium.

Caudal and lateral aspects

Following the superficial fascia around from the medial to caudal aspects, the attachment between the superficial and deep fascial layers begins to differ noticeably. Over the position of the flexor carpi ulnaris (FCU), the superficial fascia thins and becomes much closer and more limited in terms of the relative amount of sliding possible between the two layers (**Figs. 4.17–4.19**). With careful dissection, it can still be isolated over most of the caudal and lateral aspects; however, areas where the layers fuse or become integrated along with traversing nerve fibres are not uncommon. These areas are better shown than described in **Figs. 4.20–4.23**.

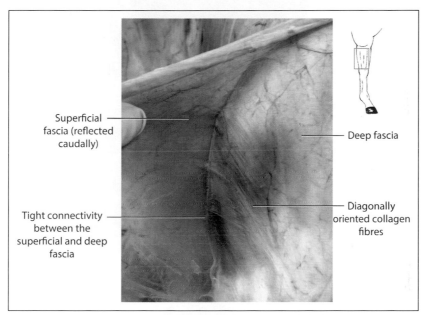

Fig. 4.17 **Connectivity between the superficial and deep fascia over the mediocaudal aspect of the left mid-antebrachium (over the flexor carpi ulnaris muscle).**

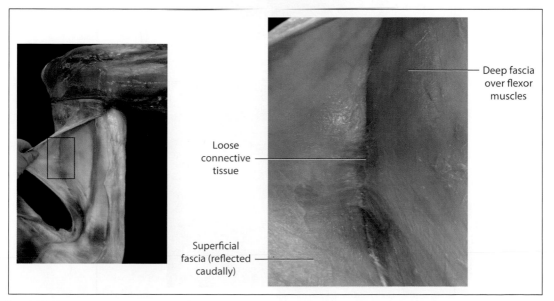

Fig. 4.18 **Loose connective tissue between the superficial and deep fascia over the caudomedial aspect of the antebrachium.**

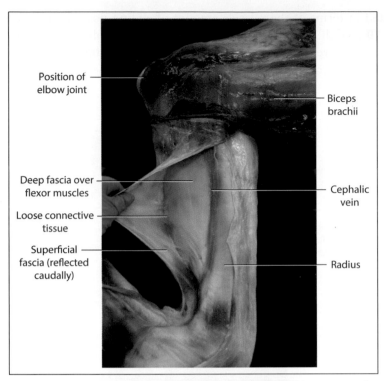

Fig. 4.19 Medial aspect of the left antebrachium with the superficial fascia severed and reflected caudally.

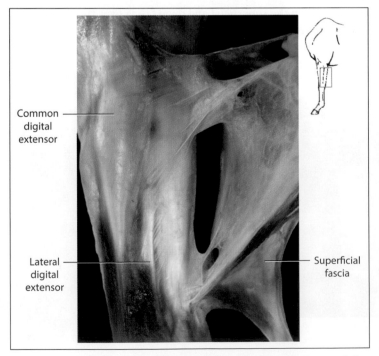

Fig. 4.20 Points of fusion between the superficial and deep fascia over the caudolateral aspect of the left antebrachium.

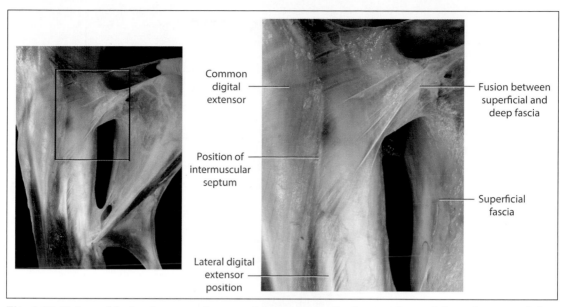

Fig. 4.21 Points of fusion between the superficial and deep fascia over the caudolateral aspect of the left antebrachium.

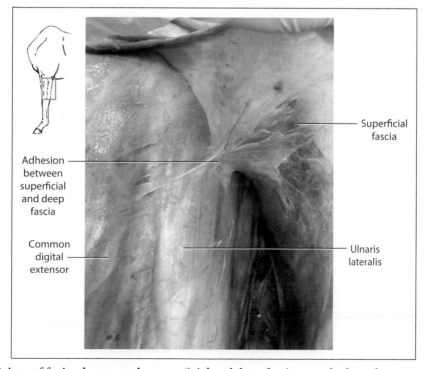

Fig. 4.22 Points of fusion between the superficial and deep fascia over the lateral aspect of the proximal antebrachium (left forelimb).

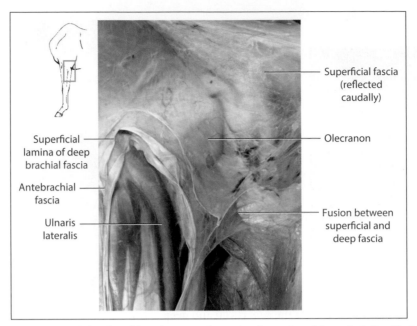

Fig. 4.23 **Lateral aspect of the distal brachium and proximal antebrachium (left forelimb).**

The final noteworthy characteristic of the superficial fascia relates to its connectivity on the craniomedial aspect of the proximal forelimb where the pectoralis transversus meets the ECR. Here, the superficial fascia is intimately connected with the overlying skin (**Fig. 4.24**). It is also intricately connected to the underlying deep fascia through a thickened tendon-like band

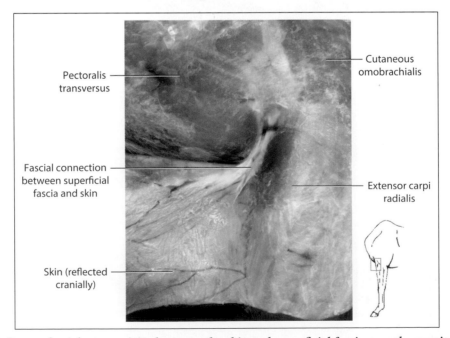

Fig. 4.24 **Strong fascial connectivity between the skin and superficial fascia over the proximal extensor carpi radialis and pectoralis transversus.**

which has boundaries that are difficult to discern due to the intimate contact between the layers (**Figs. 4.25** and **4.26**). In addition to this, the superficial fascia of this area has another two unique features. Firstly, it is joined to the underlying deep fascia through an abundance of adipose tissue, which is not encountered in any other regions of the antebrachium (**Fig. 4.27**). Secondly, it has a noticeably higher degree of elasticity than that observed over the rest of the antebrachium. This is demonstrated in **Video 7.1 (clip 1)**.

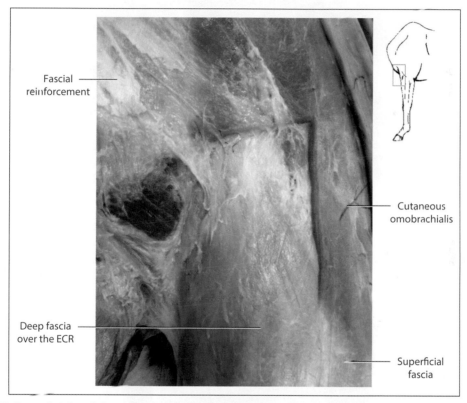

Fascial reinforcement

Cutaneous omobrachialis

Deep fascia over the ECR

Superficial fascia

Fig. 4.25 **Superficial and deep fascia over the lateral aspect of the left proximal antebrachium and brachium (the distal half of the cutaneous omobrachialis has been severed; its cranial half has been reflected dorsally).**

Locomotory efficiency

There is a high degree of stretch in the superficial fascia overlying this area of the proximal end of the ECR where it meets the pectoralis transversus muscle. This elasticity potentially contributes to the catapulting mechanism of the forelimb. Through stance, the carpus is extended by the ground reaction forces acting on the limb and tension in the lacertus fibrosus (caused by stretching of the biceps) (Wilson, Watson, & Lichtwark, 2003). Release of the ground reaction force allows recoil of the biceps and release of elastic energy which propels the forelimb forward. The increased elasticity of the fascia in this area, and its connectivity to fascia of the brachium, perhaps contributes a small amount to this elastic recoil mechanism through elbow extension and consequent stretching of this fascia. Admittedly, its effect would be minimal in comparison to the larger musculotendinous units at play here; however it is not unreasonable to conclude that it may be significant in fine tuning and coordinating the movements of the brachial and antebrachial regions of the forelimb.

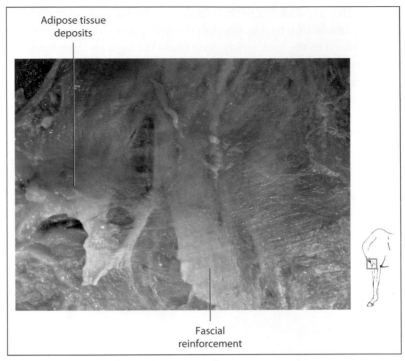

Fig. 4.26 Enforcement of the superficial fascia. Forms an attachment to the deep fascia over the dorsolateral aspect of the proximal antebrachium (fascia has been reflected dorsally).

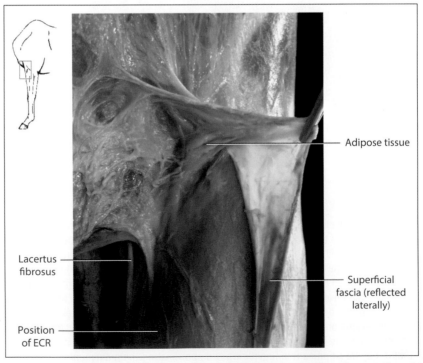

Fig. 4.27 Dorsolateral aspect of the left proximal antebrachium where the antebrachial fascia transitions into the brachial fascia.

DEEP FASCIA

Generally, the deep fascia of the forearm (antebrachial fascia) is a thick aponeurotic sheet encasing and compartmentalising the muscles of the antebrachium. It has a very limited degree of stretch and has a much more defined arrangement of fibres in comparison to the superficial fascia. In the middle third of the antebrachium, the antebrachial fascia can be followed from its attachment on the medial surface of the radius around the entire antebrachium, disregarding the intermuscular septa it gives rise to. These intermuscular septa, their attachments, and the fascial compartments formed as a consequence, are described in the following, along with how the fascia is organised in the distal third of the antebrachium to create tendon sheaths and incorporate with ligaments and fascia supporting the carpus.

Cranial compartment

The antebrachial fascia over the cranial aspect of the forearm envelops the ECR and comprises a single thick, aponeurotic sheet of connective tissue from which thinner and more membranous sheets arise. In the proximal third, the thick aponeurotic sheet has a cross-hatched fibre arrangement (proximo-distal/cranio-caudal orientation) over the insertion point of the lacertus fibrosus and over the medial aspect of the radius (**Fig. 4.28**). This fibre arrangement continues over most of the ECR surface (**Fig. 4.29**); however, distal to the lacertus fibrosus insertion and along the medial surface of the radius, it gradually fades so that a mostly vertical arrangement of fibres can be seen in the mid antebrachial region (**Fig. 4.30**). Immediately proximal to the carpus, the fibres comprising the antebrachial fascia once again became cross-hatched as shown in **Fig. 4.31**.

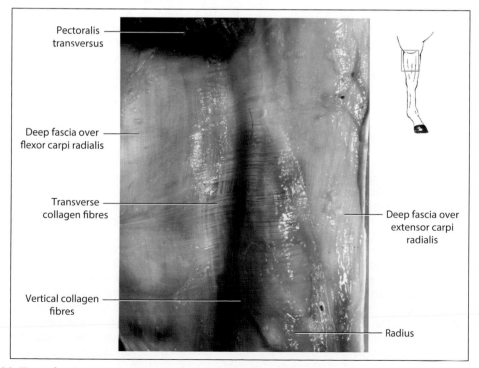

Fig. 4.28 Deep fascia spanning across the medial aspect of the left proximal antebrachium, immediately distal to the insertion of the pectoralis transversus muscle.

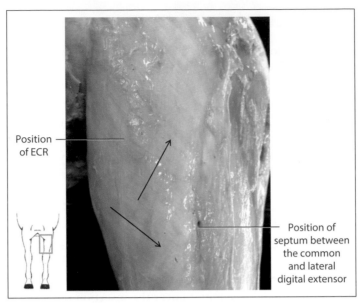

Position of ECR

Position of septum between the common and lateral digital extensor

Fig. 4.29 Antebrachial fascia over the craniolateral aspect of the left proximal antebrachium. Arrows illustrate cross-hatched fibre orientation of fascia.

Relationship between bone strain and fascial architecture

The basic principles of material design suggest that careful consideration of the fascial fibre orientation may provide a simple indication of how forces and strains are managed during weight-bearing and locomotion (Dyer, Lassila, Jokinen, & Vallittu, 2004; Rathnakar & Shivanand, 2013). In fact, a study looking at the functional construction of the fascial system in the lower limb of man found that a relationship exists between bone strain and fascial design which implies a prominent role of fascia in the management of functional strains (Gerlach & Lierse, 1990). Due to a misplaced centre of gravity in the lower limb of man, the femoral shaft is subjected to bending strains along its medial axis and tensile strains along its lateral axis (Pauwels, 1948). Gerlach and Lierse (1990) found that it was along the lateral axis of the femur where the strongest parts of the lower limb connective tissue system were located. Hence, it was concluded that the strong longitudinal fibres of both the iliotibial tract and the intermuscular septa over the lateral aspect of the leg create a tension band effect which ultimately reduces the stresses exerted on the femoral shaft through bending.

In the equine antebrachium, it is proposed here that a similar relationship between bone strain and fascial construction is present. Not unlike the femur in man, the radius of the equine forelimb is subject to bending when under load due to the natural curvature of the bone (Biewener, 1983). Tensile strains which result from this bending are greatest on the cranial and craniolateral aspects of the radius in the proximal and midshaft regions, whilst compressive strains are greatest on the caudal and medial cortices (Schneider, Milne, Gabel, Groom, & Bramlage, 1982). Our findings showed that, over the craniolateral aspect, the fibres comprising the antebrachial fascia covering the CDE in the proximal and mid regions of the forearm were arranged in a mostly longitudinal direction. This suggests that the antebrachial fascia of the forearm may act similarly to that of the lower limb in man by creating a tension band effect which reduces the amount of radial bending and the consequent stresses exerted on the bone. In addition to this, two strong intermuscular septa attach along the craniolateral aspect of the radius either side of the CDE. The nature of these septa as opposed to those described on the caudal aspect (created by thinner, more membranous fascial extensions) further supports this idea. The attachment of such thick, inelastic sheets to the periosteal surface of the bone creates a rigid system between the bone, fascia and muscles, thereby contributing to the tension band effect proposed above.

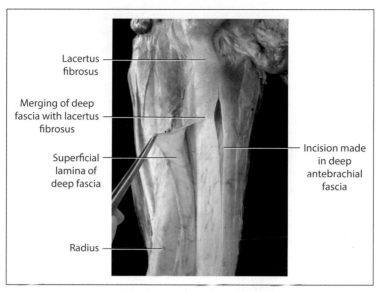

Fig. 4.30 Craniomedial aspect of left antebrachium.

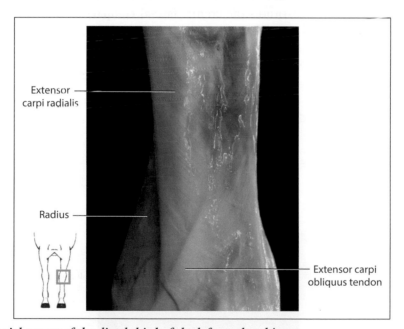

Fig. 4.31 Cranial aspect of the distal third of the left antebrachium.

Bone strain in the distal antebrachium

A small degree of compressive strain occurs in the distal region of the radius; however the most prominent strains present are torsional (Schneider et al., 1982). In parallel with these findings, the fascia in the distal region of the radius (on all aspects) has a distinct cross hatched fibre arrangement with fibres running in an oblique direction. Such an arrangement provides strong resistance to twisting forces that are acting on the antebrachium by restricting the degree of stretch possible in more than one direction.

The lacertus fibrosus itself integrates with the deep fascia and, through its connection with the biceps brachii, provides a continuous pathway between the myofascia of the brachium and antebrachium. Distal to the lacertus fibrosus insertion, the antebrachial fascia gives rise (on its superficial surface) to a thin fascial sheet that is of similar thickness and fibre arrangement to the overlying superficial fascia (**Fig. 4.30**). This layer merges distally with the antebrachial fascia at the musculotendinous junction of the ECR and laterally at the juncture of the ECR and the common digital extensor (CDE) muscles. Medially, it attaches to the cranial surface of the radius.

In the distal third of the antebrachium, yet another thin layer is present which arises from the deep surface of the aponeurotic fascial layer. This layer is closely associated with the ECR (**Fig. 4.32**) and continues distally to form the ECR tendon sheath in the region of the carpus. The thicker antebrachial fascia lying superficial to it thickens, becomes cross-hatched in its fibre arrangement, and transitions into the carpal extensor retinaculum. Immediately proximal to the carpus, it envelops the tendon of the extensor carpi obliquus (ECO) as shown in **Fig. 4.33**.

Following the aponeurotic layer around laterally, it detaches a sheet which invests between the caudal margin of the ECR and the cranial margin of the CDE (**Fig. 4.34**). The continuity of this intermuscular septum on the underside of the ECR creates an isolated pocket for the ECR and therefore constitutes the cranial fascial compartment of the antebrachium. Importantly, the antebrachial fascia is not separate from the ECR epimysium the whole way around. In the middle third of the radius, along the cranial, lateral and caudal surfaces of the ECR, the antebrachial fascia can be easily separated from the ECR epimysial fascia. However, in the proximal third of the antebrachium and along the medial surface in the middle third of the antebrachium, the thick, inelastic antebrachial fascia and epimysial fascia of the ECR muscle are strongly integrated.

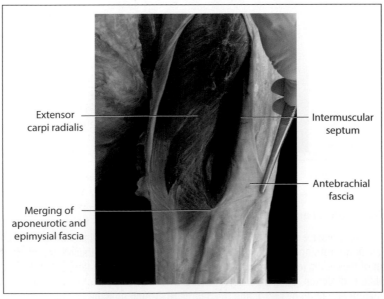

Extensor carpi radialis

Intermuscular septum

Antebrachial fascia

Merging of aponeurotic and epimysial fascia

Fig. 4.32 Proximal two-thirds of the left antebrachium (lateral aspect). Antebrachial fascia has been peeled back cranially and caudally to reveal underlying muscle.

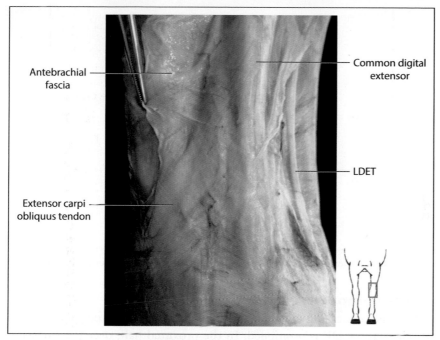

Antebrachial fascia

Common digital extensor

LDET

Extensor carpi obliquus tendon

Fig. 4.33 Distal third of the left antebrachium (craniolateral aspect). Superficial fascia has been removed.

Carpal fascia fibre orientation

Distal to the radius, the cross hatched fibre arrangement continued into the carpal region. Forces acting on the carpus have not been clearly demonstrated in the literature; however, the cross-hatched arrangement of fibres over the carpus suggests that there is a resistance to torsional strain that facilitates the action of the carpal ligaments and perhaps reduces the amount of strain they are subjected to. It has been suggested that the collateral, dorsal and palmar ligaments of the carpus are together spirally arranged so that they are tensed during axial rotation of the limb (Kadletz, 1932). Hence, the oblique cross-hatched arrangement of the carpal fascial fibres would appear to provide additional resistance to the torsional strains that result from such rotation.

Antebrachial compartments

In a clinical setting, the most useful implications of knowing the arrangement of the antebrachial fascial compartments would appear to be in the treatment, management and prevention of antebrachial compartment syndrome. However, compartment syndrome is very rarely encountered in the forelimb of horses and there have only been a few cases reported in the literature (Lindsay, McDonnell, & Bignall, 1980; Norman, Williams, Dodman, & Kraus, 1989; Sullins, Heath, Turner, & Stashak, 1987; Wallace, 1996) for which the existing descriptions of fascial compartments (although undetailed and inconsistent) were sufficient to direct treatment. Therefore, it is argued here that the importance of understanding the construction of the antebrachial fascia relates instead to how the tensional distribution of forces through the fascial network may facilitate biomechanical efficiency and load management throughout the forelimb.

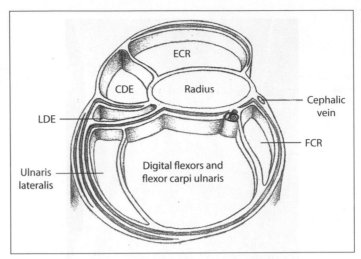

Fig. 4.34 Fascial compartments formed in the mid region of the left antebrachium.

Craniolateral compartment

The antebrachial fascia encasing the ECR on the cranial aspect is continuous over the craniolateral aspect where the CDE is positioned. In the proximal half, over the surface of the CDE muscle, it has a mostly vertical arrangement of fibres with smaller diagonally oriented fibres crossing it in a caudoproximal direction (**Fig. 4.35**). In the distal half of the antebrachium, a more cross hatched arrangement is observed. This continues over the carpus to form the extensor and flexor retinacula (**Fig. 4.36**).

As already described, the antebrachial fascia over the ECR gives rise to an intermuscular septum between the CDE and the ECR along the craniolateral aspect of the radius (**Fig. 4.34**). A second septum also invests along the caudal border of the CDE and, in this way, the craniolateral

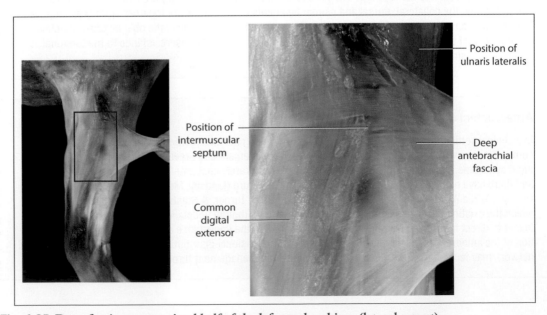

Fig. 4.35 Deep fascia over proximal half of the left antebrachium (lateral aspect).

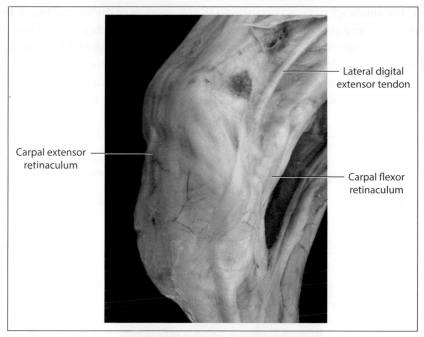

Fig. 4.36 **Fascia comprising the carpal flexor and extensor retinacula in the left forelimb.**

fascial compartment of the antebrachium is formed. An incision made in the antebrachial fascia along the middle length of the CDE reveals it to be easily separated from the epimysial fascia covering the craniolateral surface of the muscle; however, there is strong adherence between these two fascial layers on the cranial border of the CDE in the proximal third, and along the entire caudal length of the muscle belly (**Figs. 4.34** and **4.37**).

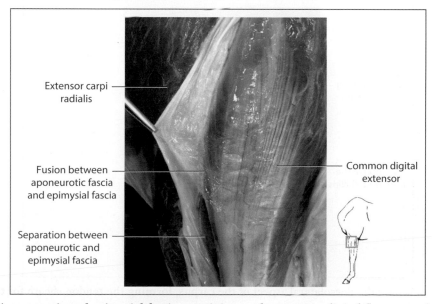

Fig. 4.37 **Aponeurotic and epimysial fascia pertaining to the common digital flexor muscle.**

Proximally, the antebrachial fascia over the CDE continues over the triceps lateral head, thereby forming a direct continuation of fascia between the brachium and antebrachium. Distal to the CDE muscle it continues as the carpal fascia and forms the dorsal wall of the CDE tendon sheath. The proximal boundary of this sheath and its remaining walls are formed from the epimysial fascia of the CDE muscle which continues distal to the musculotendinous junction and integrates with the overlying antebrachial fascia as shown in **Figs. 4.38** and **4.39**. In addition to this, the caudal wall of the

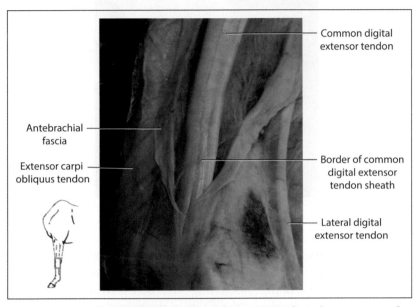

Fig. 4.38 Fascia comprising the proximal border of the common digital extensor tendon sheath in the left forelimb.

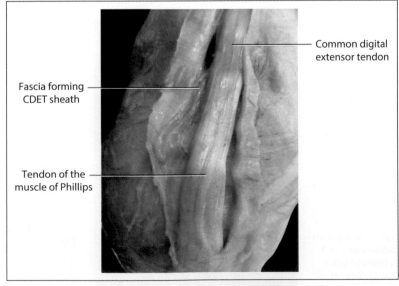

Fig. 4.39 Fascia over the dorsolateral aspect of the carpus, forming the tendon sheath for the common digital extensor tendon.

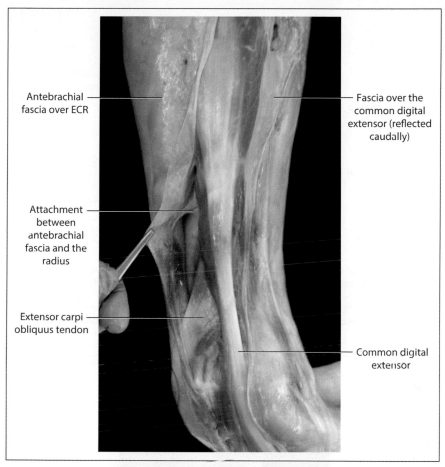

Antebrachial fascia over ECR

Fascia over the common digital extensor (reflected caudally)

Attachment between antebrachial fascia and the radius

Extensor carpi obliquus tendon

Common digital extensor

Fig. 4.40 **Craniolateral aspect of the distal half of the left antebrachium and carpus.**

tendon sheath separates the CDE from the underlying ECO. The ECO itself is strongly adhered to the periosteal surface of the radius and its tendon is intricately encased within the antebrachial fascia. This relationship is best demonstrated in **Fig. 4.40**.

Lateral compartment

The antebrachial fascia enveloping the lateral digital extensor (LDE) muscle is not a direct continuation of the antebrachial fascia extending around from the CDE muscle. Instead, it exists as a separate layer which envelops the muscle and continues over the surface of the ulnaris lateralis (**Fig. 4.34**). The fascia extending around from the CDE has a single point of attachment to the fascia of the LDE at a point slightly distal to the level of the olecranon. Aside from this, the two fascial layers remain separate over the cranial surface of the LDE along the proximal two-thirds of the antebrachium. In the distal third, the two adjoining surfaces attach as shown in **Figs. 4.41** and **4.42**.

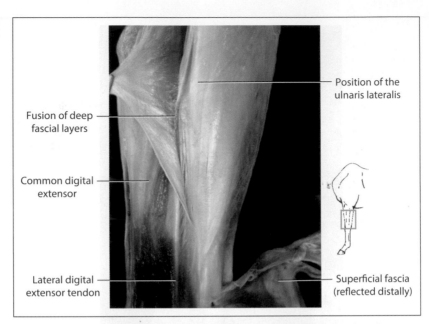

Fig. 4.41 Fusion of deep fascial layers over the lateral aspect of the left antebrachium.

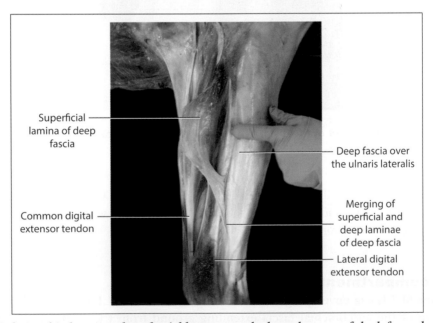

Fig. 4.42 Relationship between deep fascial layers over the lateral aspect of the left antebrachium.

The fascia of the lateral compartment comprises a very small area comparative to the other antebrachial compartments. Its most distinctive feature is the alignment of collagen fibres proximal to the carpus over the lateral digital extensor tendon (LDET) (**Figs. 4.43–4.45**). Here, fibres are arranged caudodistally and the fascia becomes continuous with the carpal flexor retinaculum and the fascia over the ulnaris lateralis (**Fig. 4.41**).

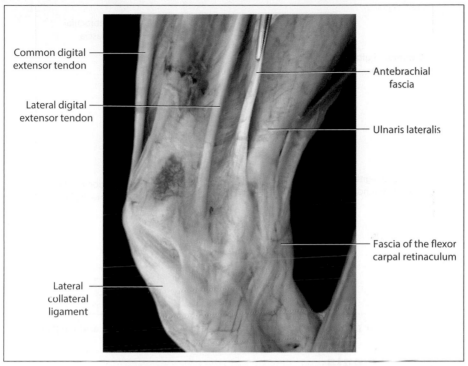

Common digital extensor tendon

Lateral digital extensor tendon

Lateral collateral ligament

Antebrachial fascia

Ulnaris lateralis

Fascia of the flexor carpal retinaculum

Fig. 4.43 Fascia of the left distal antebrachium and carpus.

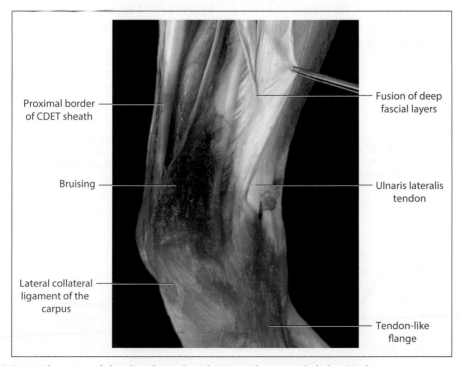

Proximal border of CDET sheath

Bruising

Lateral collateral ligament of the carpus

Fusion of deep fascial layers

Ulnaris lateralis tendon

Tendon-like flange

Fig. 4.44 Lateral aspect of the distal antebrachium and carpus (left forelimb).

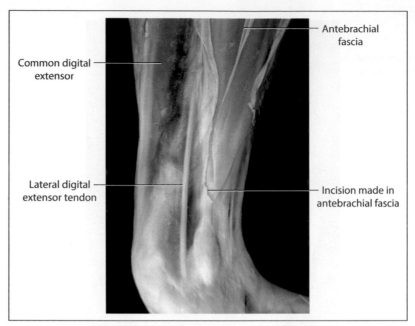

Fig. 4.45 Deep fascia over the lateral aspect of the left distal antebrachium and carpus.

Caudal compartments

The antebrachial fascia on the lateral and caudolateral aspects of the antebrachium is made complicated by the detachment and fusion of several layers. Over the caudolateral aspect, where the ulnaris lateralis is situated, two layers of fascia can be isolated. The most superficial of these, as briefly alluded to above, is a continuation of the antebrachial fascia extending from the CDE muscle (**Figs. 4.41**, **4.42** and **4.46**).

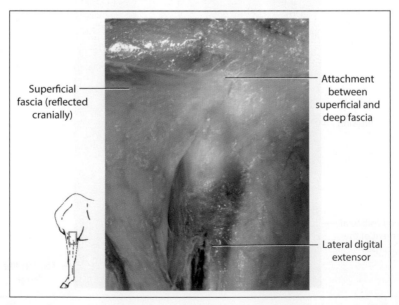

Fig. 4.46 Attachment between superficial and deep fascia over the lateral aspect of the proximal antebrachium.

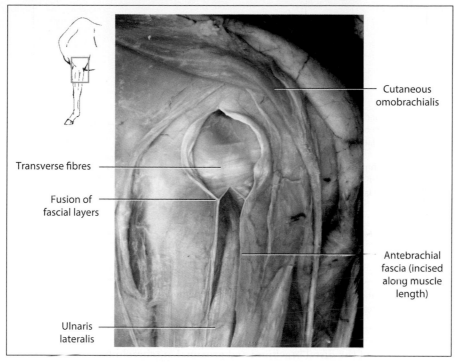

Cutaneous omobrachialis

Transverse fibres

Fusion of fascial layers

Antebrachial fascia (incised along muscle length)

Ulnaris lateralis

Fig. 4.47 **Caudolateral aspect of the left proximal antebrachium.**

Following this fascial layer around, it adopts a diagonally oriented fibre arrangement directed towards the olecranon. It is along this diagonal line that it eventually merges with the second, deeper, layer of aponeurotic fascia over the caudolateral aspect (**Figs. 4.34, 4.42** and **4.44**). This second layer of aponeurotic fascia encases the LDE and extends around the caudal to medial aspects of the antebrachium where it attaches to the medial surface of the radius. Hence, it encloses all muscles on the flexor surface of the radius (**Fig. 4.34**). At the most proximal point of the caudolateral aspect, this second layer detaches yet another small slip of fascia which displays strong, inelastic horizontal fibres crossing from the lateral epicondyle of the humerus to the olecranon of the ulna (**Figs. 4.47** and **4.48**). This creates a small pocket of space over the proximal end of the ulnaris lateralis.

To now consider the fibre orientation of the aponeurotic fascia spanning the flexor aspect; there is no constant, regular arrangement of fibres across the lateral to medial aspects nor along the proximodistal direction. Over the surface of the ulnaris lateralis, the fibres comprising the antebrachial fascia have a grossly observable proximodistal alignment (**Fig. 4.41**); however, the antebrachial fascia adopts a prominent cross-hatched fibre arrangement in the proximal third as it approaches the olecranon and becomes continuous with the brachial fascia (**Figs. 4.42** and **4.49**). **Figs. 4.50** and **4.51** demonstrate the varying fibre orientation over the caudal and caudomedial aspects of the antebrachium. A more consistent diagonal orientation occurs over the medial aspect (**Figs. 4.52** and **4.53**) distal to the TFA. Deep to the TFA however, over the medial and caudomedial aspects of the proximal antebrachium, the aponeurotic fascia has a distinctive arrangement of thick, inelastic fibres which form an obtuse 'V' orientation (**Figs 4.11** and **4.12**).

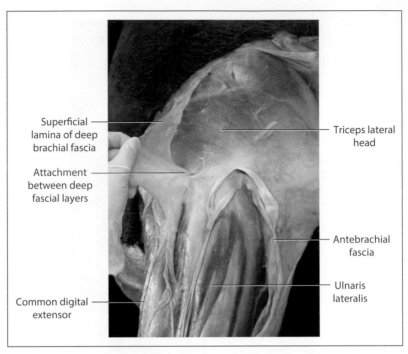

Superficial lamina of deep brachial fascia

Attachment between deep fascial layers

Common digital extensor

Triceps lateral head

Antebrachial fascia

Ulnaris lateralis

Fig. 4.48 Lateral aspect of the distal brachium and proximal antebrachium.

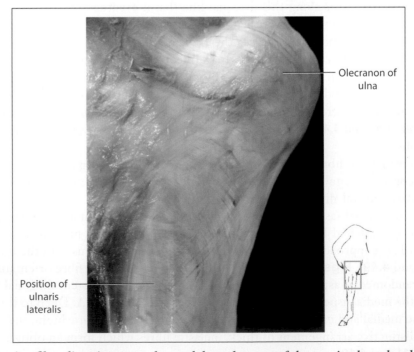

Olecranon of ulna

Position of ulnaris lateralis

Fig. 4.49 Varying fibre directions over the caudolateral aspect of the proximal antebrachium.

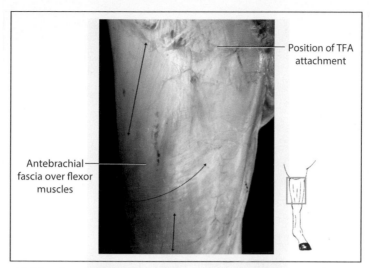

Fig. 4.50 Antebrachial fascia on the caudomedial aspect of the left antebrachium. Arrows illustrate varying fibre directions.

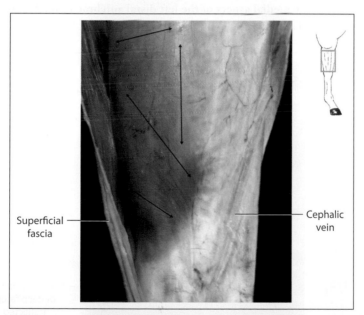

Fig. 4.51 Antebrachial fascia over the caudomedial aspect of the left distal antebrachium. Arrows illustrate varying fibre orientation.

Fibre orientation

Over the caudal aspect of the antebrachium, this varied arrangement of fibres suggests a more circumferential tension direction around the antebrachium and a tensional resistance to torsional strains. In relation to the skeletal structures of the antebrachium, it has been described how the fixed position of the radius and ulna does not allow for twisting forces (Badoux, 1974) and it has further been shown that the radius undergoes a consistent loading regime throughout locomotion (Biewener, 1983). Hence, the fibre orientation of the antebrachial fascia over the caudal aspect may facilitate resistance to torsional strains which in turn helps maintain a consistent loading pattern within the antebrachium.

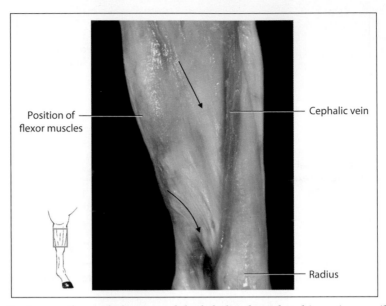

Fig. 4.52 Deep fascia over the medial aspect of the left distal antebrachium. Arrows illustrate predominant direction of collagen fibres.

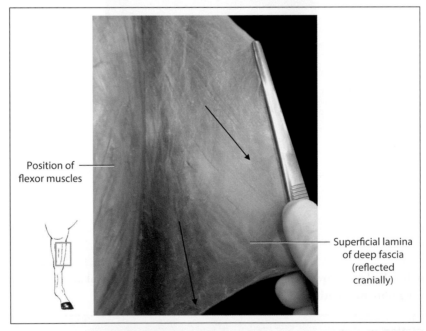

Fig. 4.53 Fibre direction of superficial lamina of deep fascia over the caudomedial aspect of the proximal to mid regions of the antebrachium. Arrows show varying fibre direction.

There are three more prominent features of this aponeurotic layer to be described. The first is that proximally along the caudal aspect it envelops the ulnar head of the deep digital flexor muscle. In this way, it links the aponeurotic fascia with the more membranous compartmentalising fascia which is described in the following (**Figs. 4.54** and **4.55**). The second is that distal and slightly medial to the ulnar head of the deep digital flexor muscle it gives rise to a thin tendinous band which

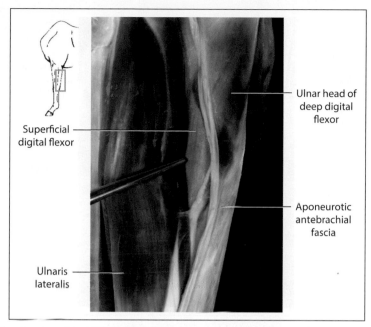

Fig. 4.54 Deep fascia over the caudolateral aspect of the proximal to mid regions of the left antebrachium.

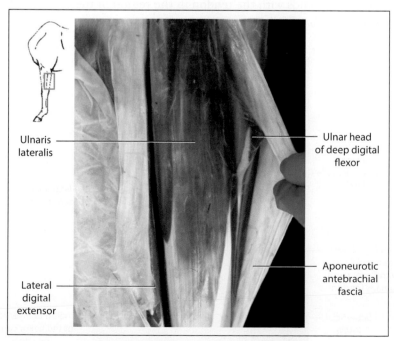

Fig. 4.55 Deep fascia over the caudolateral aspect of the proximal to mid regions of the left antebrachium.

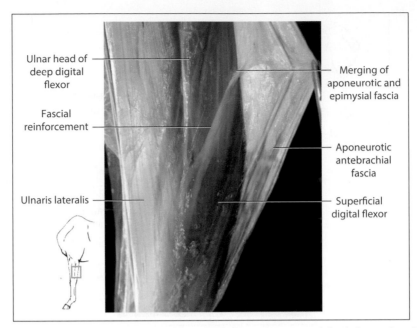

Fig. 4.56 **Aponeurotic and epimysial fascial layers in the mid region of the left antebrachium (caudolateral aspect).**

integrates with the fascia over the superficial digital flexor muscle as well as the tendon of the ulnaris lateralis muscle (**Fig. 4.56**). Finally, it is a direct continuation of the carpal flexor and extensor retinaculi. In some cases, this fascia forms tendon sheaths (as described in the following); however, in the case of the FCU, it blends with the tendon in the region of the carpus (**Figs. 4.57–4.60**) (see *carpal retinacula and tendon sheaths*).

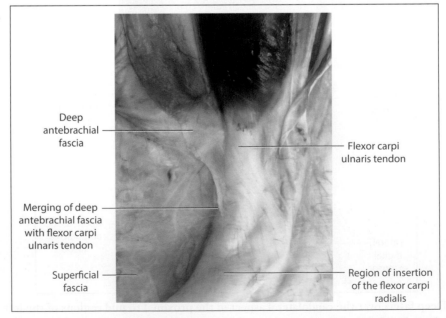

Fig. 4.57 **Relationship between fascial layers over the caudal aspect of the left distal antebrachium.**

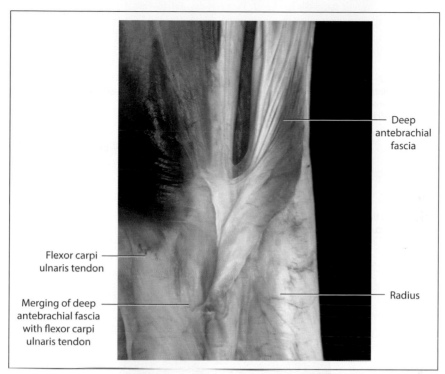

Fig. 4.58 Relationship between fascial layers over the caudomedial aspect of the left distal antebrachium.

Carpal Stability

The equine forelimb is supported against dorsiflexion when standing, walking, running or landing from a jump by not only the flexor muscles and their derived tendons, but also by the structures acting on the accessory carpal bone. The fascia covering the caudal aspect of the antebrachium is continuous with the carpal flexor retinaculum and hence strongly attached to the accessory carpal bone. This connectivity suggests that fascial tension over the caudal aspect of the antebrachium contributes to carpal stability when the limb is under load and may lessen the output required from the flexor muscles themselves. Harrison et al. (2012) found that the flexor muscles were activated from late swing phase through to early stance phase which is when the most resistance to carpal hyperextension is needed due to the interaction of load and ground reaction forces acting on the limb. Therefore, tension in the antebrachial fascia may be sufficient at mid to late stance to prevent hyperextension of the carpus when the limb is still under load whilst minimising the energy expenditure from active muscle contraction.

In addition to this, it is likely that the antebrachial fascia further contributes to carpal joint position and stability through the continuation it has with the collateral ligaments and the attachments it forms with the joint capsule. Although previous works have demonstrated clear and distinct carpal ligaments (Barone, 2010; Dyce et al., 2002; Nickel et al., 1986), investigation of the fascia demonstrates a very intimate connectivity between the fascia and collateral carpal ligaments which prevents isolation of these ligaments. Zschokke (1892) suggested that the interlocking wedge arrangement of the carpus enables transfer of sudden forces from the carpal bones to the elastic ligaments supporting the bones. Extending on this idea, it is proposed here that tensional strains acting on the carpus are redirected not only through the carpal ligaments, but also through the integrated fascia which extends proximally into the antebrachium, and distally into the metacarpus.

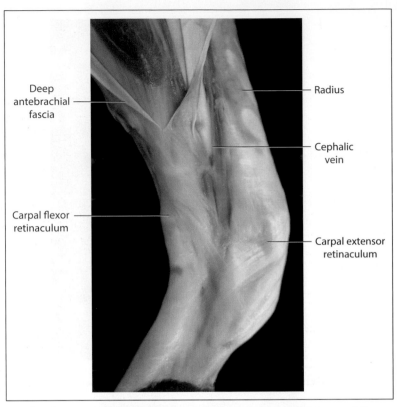

Fig. 4.59 Relationship between deep antebrachial fascia and fascia of the carpal flexor and extensor retinacula as seen on the medial aspect (left forelimb).

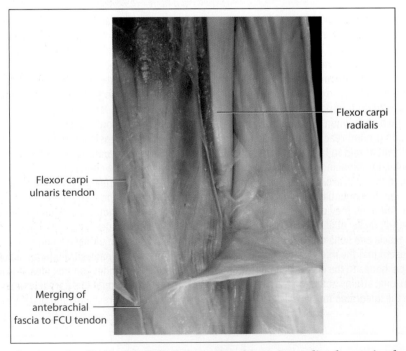

Fig. 4.60 Deep fascia at the distal end of the left antebrachium, immediately proximal to the carpus.

The organisation of more than one fascial compartment on the caudal aspect of the antebrachium is briefly alluded to above. Unlike the compartments formed on the cranial aspect of the antebrachium, those on the caudal aspect are not formed by septa which arise from the thick aponeurotic layer of antebrachial fascia. Rather, the septa compartmentalising the flexor muscles on the caudal aspect arise from a thinner membranous layer of fascia lying deep to this (**Fig. 4.34**). This membranous fascia envelops the ulnaris lateralis. It extends over the superficial and deep surfaces of the digital flexor muscles and FCU, remaining separable from their enveloping epimysial fasciae (**Figs. 4.61–4.63**). Upon reaching the FCR, it becomes integrated with the muscle and forms yet another intermuscular septum between the FCR and FCU (**Fig. 4.64**). In this way, caudolateral, caudal and caudomedial compartments are formed.

Each of these compartments remains attached to the radial periosteal surface mostly via loose connective tissue. The schematic in **Fig. 4.34** illustrates how an extension of fascia from the FCR ensheathes the median nerve and vessels and forms a single direct attachment to the caudomedial surface of the radius.

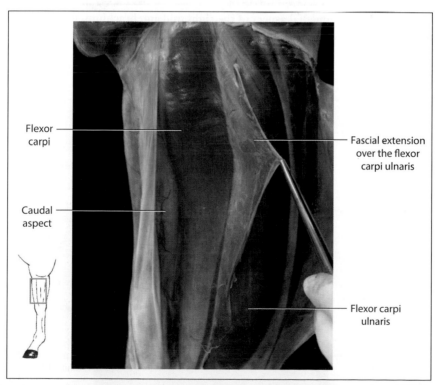

Flexor carpi

Caudal aspect

Fascial extension over the flexor carpi ulnaris

Flexor carpi ulnaris

Fig. 4.61 Fascia over the caudomedial aspect of the right mid antebrachium, demonstrating deep lamina of deep fascia.

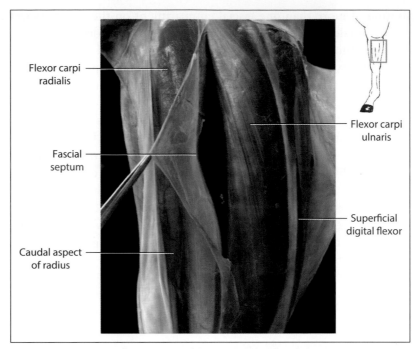

Flexor carpi
radialis

Fascial
septum

Caudal aspect
of radius

Flexor carpi
ulnaris

Superficial
digital flexor

Fig. 4.62 Fascia over the caudomedial aspect of the right mid antebrachium, demonstrating the septum between the flexor carpi radialis and flexor carpi ulnaris.

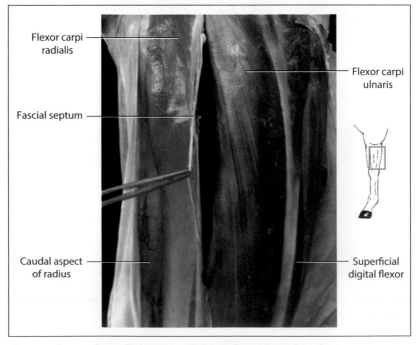

Flexor carpi
radialis

Fascial septum

Caudal aspect
of radius

Flexor carpi
ulnaris

Superficial
digital flexor

Fig. 4.63 Fascia over the caudomedial aspect of the right mid antebrachium.

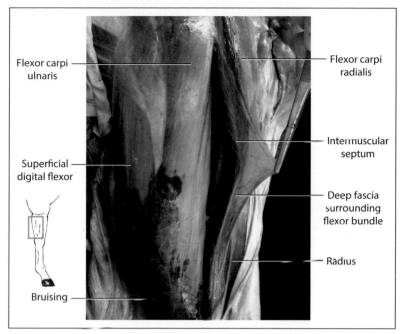

Fig. 4.64 Caudomedial aspect of the antebrachium with the superficial fascia removed and the antebrachial fascia peeled back.

Carpal retinacula and tendon sheaths

The carpal fascia is a direct distal extension of the antebrachial fascia. Over the dorsal aspect, it forms tendon sheaths for the ECR, CDE and ECO tendons which maintain their position with manual flexion and extension of the carpal joint. Over the flexor aspect, the carpal fascia is slightly more complicated in its arrangement due to the attachment of fascia to the accessory carpal bone, as well as the formation of the carpal flexor tendon sheath.

In relation to the common digital extensor tendon (CDET) on the dorsal aspect, the aponeurotic fascial layer in the distal third of the antebrachium continues over the carpus to form the dorsal wall of the CDE tendon sheath. At the musculotendinous junction, it gives rise to an additional thin fascial sheet which forms the deep surface of the CDET sheath (**Fig. 4.38**) and attaches along the tendon length to form a membranous extension. This extension connects to the fascia of the carpal joint capsule forming two strong points of attachment. The first is at the level of the antebrachiocarpal joint space, just above the intermediate carpal bone. A second strong point of attachment occurs over the distal end of the radius between the CDET and the ECO tendon (**Fig. 4.65**).

Medial to this, the arrangement of fascia becomes complex as a tendon sheath is formed around the ECO tendon and the ECR tendon. The tendon sheath surrounding the ECO tendon appears to be derived from the same membranous fascia running deep to the CDET but is still connected to the thick antebrachial fascia of the ECR. The ECR tendon itself is enveloped within a thin layer of fascia which forms in the distal third of the antebrachium as described earlier.

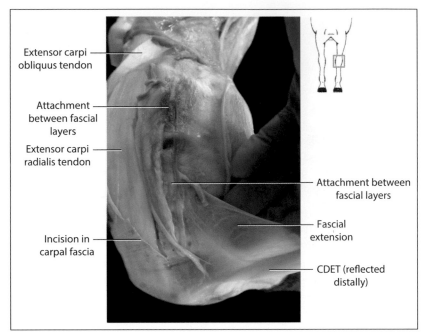

Extensor carpi
obliquus tendon

Attachment
between fascial
layers

Extensor carpi
radialis tendon

Incision in
carpal fascia

Attachment between
fascial layers

Fascial
extension

CDET (reflected
distally)

Fig. 4.65 Dorsal aspect of the antebrachium with the common digital extensor tendon peeled back distally.

Fascial continuity and functional integration across joints

Fascial continuity across limb segments suggests that there is an aspect of limb coordination and control which is dependent on the passive transmission of forces rather than being exclusively controlled by the nervous system. The continuity between the carpal ligaments and the fascia is one example of this, as is the continuation of the antebrachial fascia with the carpal flexor retinaculum and the FCU tendon. Another example is the tendon-like flange associated with the LDET. This fascial extension blends distally with the LDET in the proximal third of the metacarpus and proximally with the fascia comprising the carpal flexor retinaculum. It therefore provides a direct pathway from the dorsal aspect of the proximal phalanx (to which the LDET attaches) to the caudal aspects of the carpus and antebrachium (with which the carpal fascia is continuous). In this way, fascial tension over the caudal aspect of the antebrachium may contribute in a small way to distal forelimb extension. To further support this idea, attention is brought to studies investigating muscle function and joint positioning throughout the stride. Harrison et al. (2012) described how all muscles of the proximal forelimb are active just prior to hoof strike which is when extension of the digit is required. Active contractility of flexor muscles in the antebrachium (most particularly the ulnaris lateralis due to its position laterally) is likely to create tension in the antebrachial and carpal fascia which then translates to the LDET on the dorsal aspect of the carpus via the fascial extension described above.

This idea of muscle activity through fascial tension highlights the importance of considering and recognizing muscle activity beyond their traditionally described origins and insertions. In fact, several other relationships between the fascia and muscles of the antebrachium provide support for this idea.

In a similar way, the pectoralis transversus muscle finds insertion in the superficial fascia of the antebrachium, which continues distally as an irregularly arranged sheet into the region of the metacarpus and proximal digit. The relatively dispersed distribution of fibres comprising the majority of the superficial fascia in the antebrachium suggests an ability to respond to multidirectional loads. However, areas with a more organized, parallel arrangement of fibres imply a more direct, focused path of tension distribution. The parallel fibres aligned dorsodistally over the caudomedial aspect of the antebrachium is a prime example of this. They serve as a continuous connection between the carpal fascia and the fascia enveloping the pectoralis transversus. Hence, tensional forces distributed proximally from the digit to the dorsomedial aspect of the carpus are, in part, directed to the medial aspect of the antebrachium (and presumably to the brachium also) via the proximal connectivity of the pectoralis transversus. Considering this relationship in reverse, this fascial alignment further suggests that the action of pectoralis transversus extends beyond its distal margin and may transmit distally via contractile forces distributed through the superficial fascia.

On the lateral aspect, the carpal fascia is observed to be a direct extension of the lateral collateral ligament of the carpus, under which the LDET passes (**Figs. 4.66** and **4.67**). Although often illustrated as a distinct structure, the lateral collateral ligament cannot be isolated from the antebrachial fascia proximally, nor can it be isolated along its lateral and medial margins from the surrounding fascia comprising the carpal retinacula. Instead, it is identifiable by the change in fibre direction and the identification of surrounding structures (such as the LDET). It is directly continuous with the fascial layers described over the LDE and ulnaris lateralis muscles proximally, as well as with the tendon-like flange of the LDET. Distally this flange crosses obliquely from the caudolateral aspect of the carpus and attaches to the LDET at the base of the metacarpus (**Fig. 4.66**).

Caudomedially, the antebrachial fascia continues distally to form a tendon sheath for the FCR. The proximal boundary of this sheath is observed in the middle of the distal third of the radius (**Fig. 4.68**) whilst the distal margin of this sheath can be followed to the base of the metacarpus. Similar to the CDET, the fascia forming the proximal boundary of the FCR tendon sheath attaches to the tendon along its length thereby forming a sheet like extension within which string-like fascial reinforcements are present (**Fig. 4.68**).

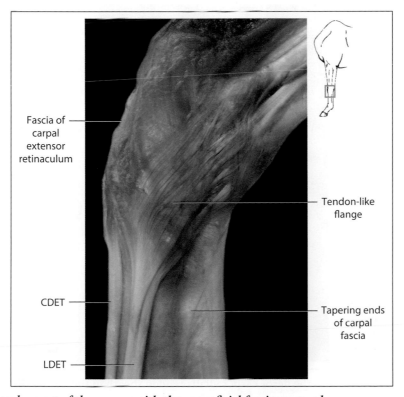

Fascia of carpal extensor retinaculum

Tendon-like flange

CDET

Tapering ends of carpal fascia

LDET

Fig. 4.66 **Lateral aspect of the carpus with the superficial fascia removed.**

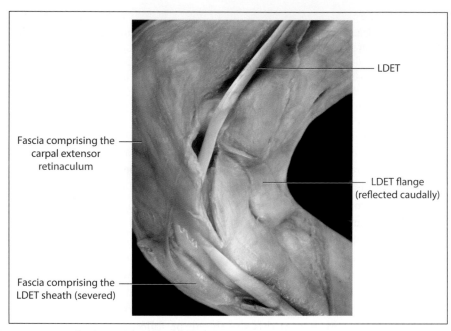

Fig. 4.67   Fascia over the lateral aspect of the left carpus and proximal metacarpus.

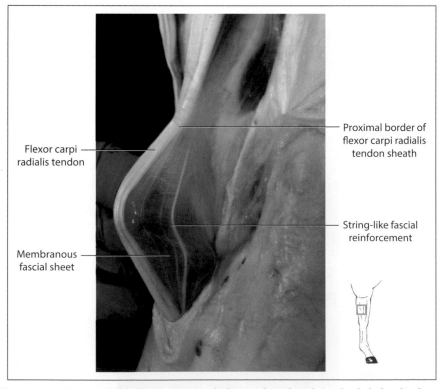

Fig. 4.68   Fascia pertaining to the flexor carpi radialis tendon sheath in the left forelimb.

The FCU is unique in this region in that no tendon sheath is formed. Instead, the antebrachial fascia blends with the tendon in the distal third of the antebrachium (**Figs. 4.57** and **4.58**) and becomes continuous with the cross hatched fibre arrangement crossing the flexor aspect of the carpus. This fibre orientation continues past the carpo-metacarpal joint and eventually fades to form the distal concave margin of the carpal flexor retinaculum.

The distal extremity of the tendon sheath surrounding the superficial and deep digital flexor tendons has been described in the previous chapter. Its proximal extremity occurs at the level of the proximal check ligament.

REFERENCES

Badoux, D. (1974). Some notes on the biomechanics of the equine antebrachium. *Z Anat Entwickl-Gesch*, *144*, 215–225.

Barone, R. (2010). *Arthrologie et Myologie* (4th ed., Vol. 2). Paris: Éditions Vigot.

Biewener, A. (1983). Bone stress in the horse forelimb during locomotion at different gaits: A comparison of two experimental methods. *Journal of Biomechanics*, *16*(8), 565–576.

Brown, N., Pandy, M., Buford, W., Kawcak, C., & McIlwraith, C. (2003). Moment arms about the carpal and metacarpophalangeal joints for flexor and extensor muscles in equine forelimbs. *American Journal of Veterinary Research*, *64*(3), 351–357.

Butcher, M., Hermanson, J., Ducharme, N., Mitchell, L., Soderholm, L., & Bertram, J. (2009). Contractile behavior of the forelimb digital flexors during steady-state locomotion in horses (*Equus caballus*): An initial test of muscle architectural hypotheses about in vivo function. *Comparative Biochemistry and Physiology Part A: Molecular & Integrative Physiology*, *152*(1), 100–114. doi:10.1016/j.cbpa.2008.09.007

Dyce, K., Sack, W., & Wensing, C. (2002). *Textbook of Veterinary Anatomy* (3rd ed.). Philadelphia, PA: W.B. Saunders.

Dyer, S., Lassila, L., Jokinen, M., & Vallittu, P. (2004). Effect of fibre position and orientation on fracture load of fibre-reinforced composite. *Dental Materials*, *20*(10), 947–955.

Gerlach, U., & Lierse, W. (1990). Functional construction of the superficial and deep fascia system of the lower limb in man. *Acta Anatomica*, *139*, 11–25.

Harrison, S. M., Whitton, R. C., King, M., Haussler, K. K., Kawcak, C. E., Stover, S. M., & Pandy, M. G. (2012). Forelimb muscle activity during equine locomotion. *Journal of Experimental Biology*, *215*(17), 2980–2991.

Hermanson, J., & Cobb, M. (1992). Four forearm flexor muscles of the horse, *Equus caballus*: Anatomy and histochemistry. *Journal of Morphology*, *212*(3), 269–280. doi:10.1002/jmor.1052120306.

Kadletz, M. (1932). *Anatomischer Atlas der Extremitätengelenke von Pferd und Hund*. Berlin: Urban & Schwarzenberg.

Lindsay, W., McDonnell, W., & Bignall, W. (1980). Equine postanesthetic forelimb lameness: intracompartmental muscle pressure changes and biomechanical patterns. *American Journal of Veterinary Research*, *41*, 1919–1924.

Nickel, R., Schummer, A., Seiferle, E., Wilkens, H., Wille, K.-H., & Frewein, J. (1986). *The Anatomy of the Domestic Mammals* (Vol. 1). Berlin: Verlag Paul Parey.

Norman, W., Williams, R., Dodman, N., & Kraus, A. (1989). Postanesthetic compartmental syndrome in a horse. *Journal of the American Veterinary Medical Association*, *195*(4), 502–504.

Pauwels, F. (1948). The principles of construction of the locomotor system: Their significance for the stressing of the tubular bones. *Z Anat EntwGesh*, *114*, 129–166.

Rathnakar, G., & Shivanand, H. (2013). Fibre orientation and its influence on the flexural strength of glass fibre and graphite fibre reinforces polymer composites. *International Journal of Innovative Research in Science, Engineering and Technology*, *2*(3), 548–552.

Schneider, R., Milne, D., Gabel, A., Groom, J., & Bramlage, L. (1982). Multidirectional in vivo strain analysis of the equine radius and tibia during dynamic loading with and without a cast. *American Journal of Veterinary Research, 43*(9), 1541–1550.

Sullins, K., Heath, R., Turner, A., & Stashak, T. (1987). Possible antebrachial flexor compartment syndrome as a cause of lameness in two horses. *Equine Veterinary Journal, 19*(2), 147–150.

Wallace, M. (1996). Compartment syndrome in a mare. *Equine Practice, 18*(3), 11–14.

Wilson, A., Watson, J., & Lichtwark, G. (2003). Biomechanics: A catapult action for rapid limb protraction. *Nature, 421*(6918), 35–36.

BIBLIOGRAPHY

Biewener, A., Thomason, J., Goodship, A., & Lanyon, L. (1983). Bone stress in the horse forelimb during locomotion at different gaits: A comparison of two experimental methods. *Journal of Biomechanics, 16*(8), 565–576.

Bradley, O. (1920). *The Topographical Anatomy of the Limbs of the Horse.* Edinburgh: W. Green & Son.

Ellenberger, W., & Baum, H. (1906). *Handbuch der Vergleichenden Anatomie der Haustiere.* Berlin: Verlag von August Hirschwald.

Paulli, S., & Sörensen, E. (1930). *Die Fascien des Pferdes.* Kopenhagen, Dänemark: Königl Tierärytliche und Landwirtschaftliche Hochschule.

Sisson, S., & Grossman, J. (1938). *The Anatomy of the Domestic Animals* (3rd ed.). Philadelphia, PA: W.B. Saunders.

von Rubeli O. (1925). Zur Anatomie und Mechanik des Karpalgelenks der Haustiere, Speziell des Pferdes. *Schweizer Archiv für Tierheilkunde, 67,* 427–432.

Zarucco, L., Taylor, K., & Stover, S. (2004). Determination of muscle architecture and fibre characteristics of the superficial and deep digital flexor muscles in the forelimbs of adult horses. *American Journal of Veterinary Research, 65*(6), 819–828.

Zschokke. (1892). *Weitere Untersuchungen über das Verhältnis der Knochenbildung.* Füssli: Zürich. [Cited by Rubeli, 1925.]

INTRODUCTION

The fascial anatomy and its functional significance in the equine distal forelimb and antebrachium has been described and discussed in the previous two chapters. How this relates functionally to the equine brachium and shoulder girdle is, at this point in time, difficult to discern due to the lack of anatomical detail available pertaining to the fascia of these two upper limb segments. Reasons as to why there have been limited investigations into the fascial anatomy of the proximal forelimb are likely related to its anatomical complexity as well as the relative impact that proximal forelimb injuries have on the racing industry. Although humeral stress fractures in racing Thoroughbreds are relatively common, their prognosis and the ability for affected horses to return to previous performance levels is quite good. Hence, their welfare and economic impact relative to that of distal forelimb injuries is much less, as is the inclination to investigate the anatomy of this area.

The problem with this is that the classical view of biomechanics relegates the connective tissue to a mere supportive role meaning that studies on injury-prone distal forelimb structures disregard the tensional distribution of forces which occurs through the connective tissue across different segments of the forelimb. It has been shown that fascia is stretched by the contraction of underlying muscles and can mechanically transmit tension at a distance. Considering that all the musculature controlling forelimb movement is proximal to the carpus, much of the action of the distal limb is almost certainly initiated in the upper limb and transmitted via fascial tension distribution to the distal forelimb. This means that the distribution of forces in the proximal forelimb most likely influences the stress, strain and functional capacity of distal forelimb joints, ligaments, tendons and bones.

The implications of the distribution and connections of the antebrachial fascia on distal forelimb movement have already been described; however, based on investigations in humans which have demonstrated the extensive continuity of the fascial system, as well as our own observations in the previous study (showing antebrachial fascia to continue proximally into the brachial region), it is suggested here that fascia of the brachium and shoulder serves as a mechanical continuum between the thorax, neck, antebrachium and distal forelimb. In humans, it has been suggested that both the thoracolumbar fascia and the fascia of the anterior region of the trunk may be implicated in the transmission of traction between the inferior and superior limbs, as well as between contralateral limbs. In horses, similar connectivity (if it exists) would have even greater implications as the forelimbs have no skeletal attachment to the axial skeleton and are instead supported by a myofascial girdle. The speed and efficiency of forelimb movement in the horse suggests that the muscles of the proximal forelimb and shoulder do not act as autonomous structures and are instead mechanically integrated through an extensive fascial network which is continuous throughout the entire limb as well as extending from the associated regions of the trunk and neck.

SUPERFICIAL FASCIA

General findings

The superficial fascia over the lateral aspect of the shoulder and brachium can be cleanly isolated from the overlying skin. It exists as a distinct layer over these regions and is continuous cranially and caudally with the superficial fascia of the neck and trunk respectively. Distally, the superficial fascia of the brachium is continuous with the superficial fascia of the antebrachium.

Similarly, the superficial fascia over the lateral aspect can also be easily isolated from the underlying deep fascial layers. There are, however, some consistent areas of stronger connectivity and attachments as described in the following. The alignment of collagen fibres comprising the superficial fascia on the lateral aspect, evident through gross observation, is largely irregular and therefore allows for a fair degree of multidirectional elasticity. The strength of its adherence to the underlying deep fascia is dependent on the length and density of the loose connective tissue fibres present between the layers and varies considerably across the shoulder. There is no obvious superficial fascia layer present on the medial aspect of the brachium.

Continuity and attachment

The most notable characteristic of the superficial fascia on the lateral aspect is that it tightly envelops the cutaneous omobrachialis muscle. This muscle covers most of the shoulder region spanning dorsoventrally from the approximate level of the scapular cartilage to the elbow joint (**Fig. 5.1**). From the dorsal margin of the cutaneous omobrachialis, the superficial fascia

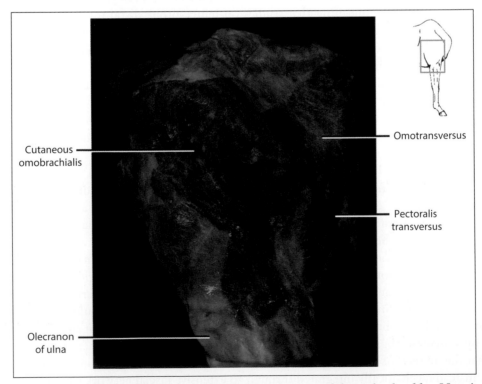

Fig. 5.1 Cutaneous omobrachialis muscle over the lateral aspect of the right shoulder. Note its continuity with the omotransversus cranially.

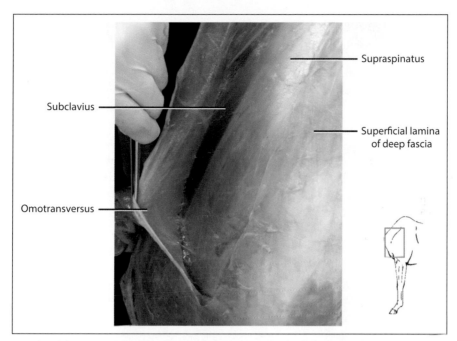

Fig. 5.2 Superficial lamina of deep fascia over the ventral half of the supraspinatus and subclavius in a left forelimb.

continues as a thin, irregular layer over the surface of the ventral half of the trapezius (which remained after removing the limb from the trunk). Here, it is very closely adhered to the fascia enveloping the ventral portion of the trapezius thoracis so that no movement can be elicited between the tissue planes.

Following the superficial fascia cranially from the position of the spine of the scapula, it can be isolated from the fascia overlying the supraspinatus (**Fig. 5.2**) and the cervical part of the trapezius. Over the dorsal quarter of the supraspinatus, the superficial fascia has a very fibrous connection to the underlying deep fascia (**Fig. 5.3**). Applying traction in the dorsal direction to the reflected superficial layer demonstrates how this dense, fibrous connective tissue serves as a direct tension distribution pathway between the superficial and deep fascial layers. In contrast, the superficial fascia over the trapezius cervicis has a much tighter connection which makes it difficult to isolate without perforating the fascia encasing the muscle (**Fig. 5.4**).

Because of its coverage over these muscles and their extension into the neck region, the superficial fascia does not continue around the cranial aspect of the shoulder to the medial aspect and is instead continuous with the superficial fascia of the base of the neck. As it courses ventrally over the omotransversus and brachiocephalicus muscles, the superficial fascia thins considerably and has a very similar connection to that observed over the trapezius cervicis. It can still, however, be detached as a delicate layer (**Figs. 5.5** and **5.6**) which invests between the ventral surface of the brachiocephalicus and the dorsal surface of the pectoralis descendens. Here, it remains detached from the brachiocephalicus, but closely envelops the pectoralis descendens, creating a friction reduced medium between the two muscles. This fascia also provides a protective encasement for the cephalic vein and becomes continuous with the superficial fascia of the antebrachium as shown in **Fig. 5.7**.

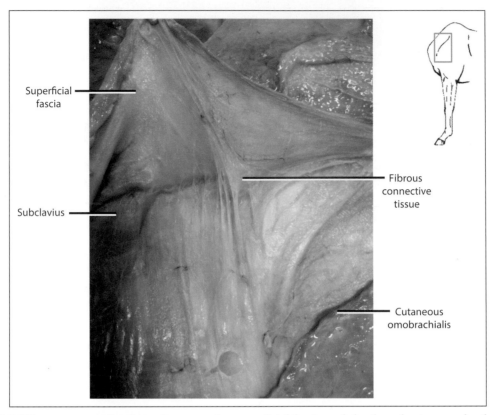

Fig. 5.3 Fibrous connective tissue between the superficial fascia and the deep fascia over the dorsal quarter of the supraspinatus and the scapula spine. The superficial fascia has been reflected dorsally (left forelimb).

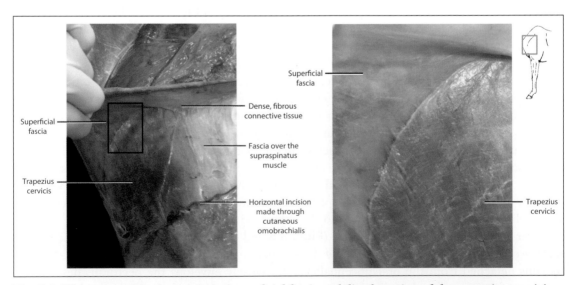

Fig. 5.4 The connectivity between the superficial fascia and distal portion of the trapezius cervicis cranial to the supraspinatus muscle (left forelimb). The superficial fascia has been severed and peeled back dorsally.

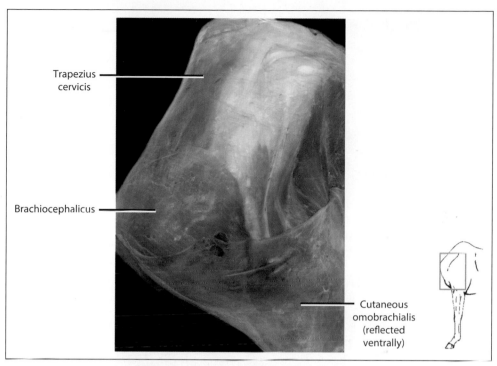

Fig. 5.5 Superficial fascia peeled back ventrally over the lateral aspect of the left shoulder.

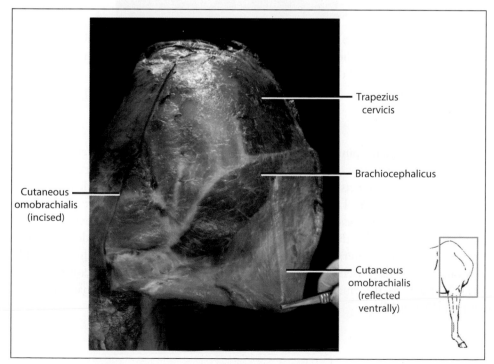

Fig. 5.6 Superficial fascia over the lateral aspect of the right brachium and shoulder.

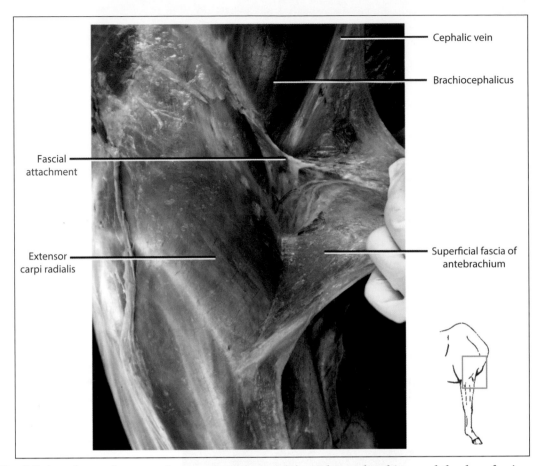

Fig. 5.7 **Attachment between the superficial fascia of the right antebrachium and the deep fascia on the cranial aspect of the antebrachium. Note the continuity between the superficial fascia of the antebrachium and brachium and the relationship it has with the cephalic vein.**

Caudal to the scapular spine, the superficial fascia encasing the cutaneous omobrachialis remains an independent layer over the deltoideus and triceps muscle. Here, a loose web-like arrangement of fibres connects the superficial and deep fascial planes with occasional fascial adhesions (**Figs. 5.8** and **5.9**). Lines along which the superficial fascia adheres to the deep fascia prevent excessive sliding of these fascial planes and occur over the juncture between: (1) the deltoideus and triceps and (2) the deltoideus and infraspinatus. A short distance dorsal to the adjoining margins of the triceps lateral and long heads, the superficial fascia on the underside of the cutaneous omobrachialis muscle detaches a separate sheet which becomes continuous with the deep fascia. In doing so, it forms a boundary that separates the interfascial space of the shoulder and brachium (**Fig. 5.10**).

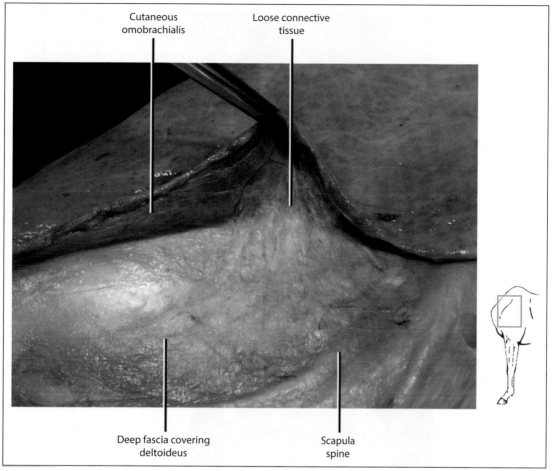

Cutaneous omobrachialis

Loose connective tissue

Deep fascia covering deltoideus

Scapula spine

Fig. 5.8 Loose connective tissue between the superficial fascia enveloping the cutaneous omobrachialis and the deep fascia over the deltoideus, caudal to the scapula spine. The superficial fascia has been reflected ventrally (left forelimb).

The role of the superficial fascia

The superficial fascia in the antebrachium and distal limb continue uninterrupted into the brachial and shoulder regions of the forelimb. The significance of this is twofold. Firstly and most obviously, it exists as an additional tissue layer which may help with the mechanical coordination of different limb segments. Secondly, its multidirectional fibre orientation suggests that it allows a certain degree of elasticity in response to various directional forces. A completely rigid system in which the deep fascia is regularly aligned would be specific in its direction of, and would be unyielding to, minor disturbances which direct forces along alternate paths. Therefore, a more elastic superficial layer provides a medium that is more capable of responding to wayward forces, thereby contributing to the overall stability of the limb and the organization of force distribution paths.

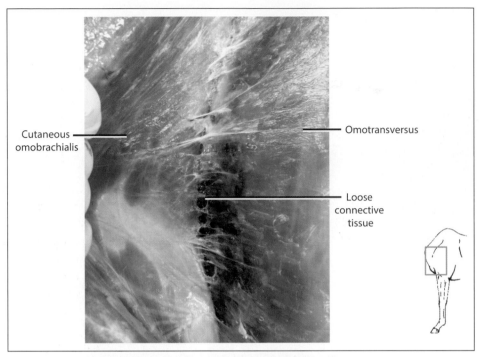

Fig. 5.9 Loose connective tissue over the cranial aspect of the left shoulder between the superficial fascia and the underlying superficial lamina of deep fascia covering the omotransversus.

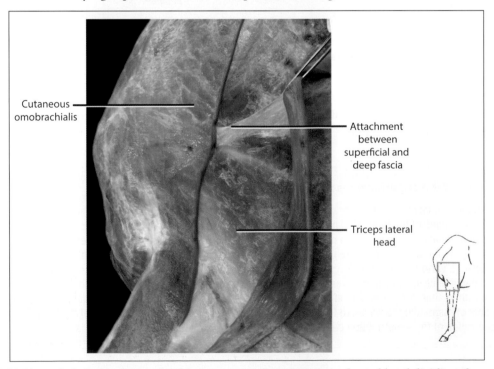

Fig. 5.10 Extended sheet of superficial fascia proximal to the triceps lateral head dividing the space between the superficial and deep fascial layers into a dorsal and ventral space. The cutaneous omobrachialis (and hence superficial fascia) has been severed along its middle length (left forelimb).

Dorsally, the cutaneous omobrachialis becomes continuous with the cutaneous trunci muscle at the caudal border of the scapula. This gives rise to extensive mechanical connectivity between the lateral aspect of the shoulder, the medial aspect of the shoulder, the trunk region, and the antebrachium. The cutaneous trunci tapers to a prominent fascial band which passes along the dorsal border of the deep pectoral muscle and inserts on the brachium. As will be described in more detail in the following, this fascial band is continuous with the fascia of the latissimus dorsi (which extends into the thorax region) as well as the teres major. In addition to this, the cutaneous trunci has a direct attachment to the fascia of the latissimus dorsi and the triceps long head at the point where they meet (**Fig. 5.11**), thereby reinforcing this association between the trunk, shoulder and brachial regions.

Two areas of distinct continuity exist between the superficial and deep fascia in the brachial region. The first occurs at the junction of the extensor carpi radialis, brachiocephalicus and pectoralis descendens (cranial aspect of proximal antebrachium and brachium). Fatty tissue is often abundant in this area (**Figs. 5.6** and **5.7**). Through this point, the superficial fascia of the brachium also becomes continuous on the craniomedial aspect with the superficial fascia of the antebrachium. The second point of continuity occurs immediately dorsal to the olecranon. This is best shown, rather than described, in **Figs. 5.12** and **5.13**. Through the attachments illustrated, the boundaries of the superficial fascia are lost around the caudal aspect of the brachium and shoulder, so that the fascial layer described as superficial on the lateral aspect, becomes directly continuous with the deep fascia enveloping the tensor fascia antebrachii (TFA) and the dorsal extension of the deep antebrachial fascia on the medial aspect. In this way, there is indistinct continuity between the superficial and deep fascial layers of the antebrachium, brachium and shoulder.

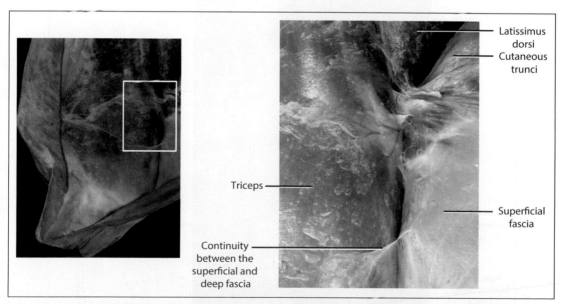

Fig. 5.11 The continuity between the superficial and deep fascia over the caudal aspect of the tricep's long head, slightly proximal to the olecranon of the ulna. Note how the cutaneous trunci is continuous with both the epimysial fascia of the latissimus dorsi as well as the superficial lamina of deep fascia over the triceps (left forelimb).

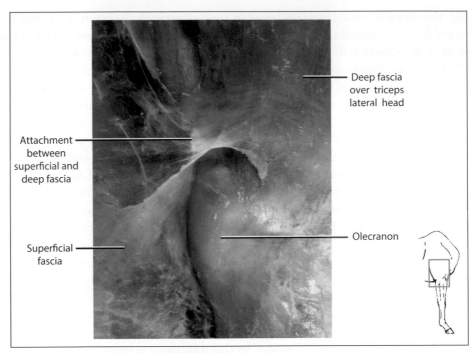

Fig. 5.12 Continuity between the superficial and deep fascia over the right elbow joint. The superficial fascia has been reflected caudally.

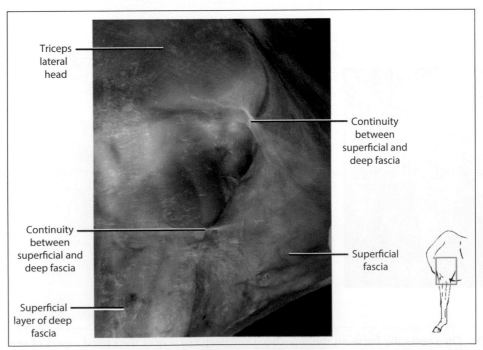

Fig. 5.13 Continuity between the superficial fascia of the brachium and antebrachium. Note the points where the superficial fascia integrates with the deep fascia along the caudal aspect of the proximal antebrachium (left forelimb).

DEEP FASCIA

General findings

The deep fascia of the brachium (fascia brachialis) and shoulder girdle (fascia omobrachialis) is interconnected and serves to mechanically link several adjoining and distant muscles. In several instances, the deep fascia integrates with the muscle fibres rather than existing as a separate overlying layer.

The deep fascia over both the lateral and medial aspects consists of two separable laminae. Lying immediately deep to the superficial fascia over the lateral aspect, a well-defined lamina (superficial lamina of the deep fascia) can be isolated which envelops the superficial shoulder muscles including the trapezius, omotransversus and brachiocephalicus muscles. The remaining muscles of the shoulder and brachium are supported by the deep lamina of the deep fascia as described in the following. The deep fascial layers over the medial aspect are made much more complicated by the brachial plexus and various axillary vessels. Once again, superficial and deep laminae are present; however, the margins of these are much less clear.

LATERAL ASPECT

Superficial lamina

This layer has a strong attachment to the protruding scapula spine and blends with the aponeurotic fascia encasing the dorsal quarter of the deltoideus. It is otherwise present as a membranous layer over most of the shoulder and brachial regions. It is most easily identified by transecting straight through the brachiocephalicus on the lateral aspect of the shoulder joint (**Figs. 5.14** and **5.15**). On either side of the scapula spine, this superficial lamina is thick and inelastic with cross-hatched fibres directed cranioventrally and dorsoventrally (**Fig. 5.16**). This cross-hatched arrangement continues ventrally

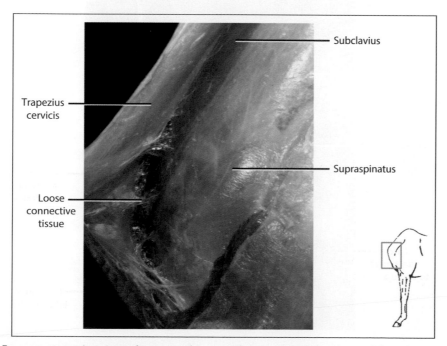

Fig. 5.14 Loose connective tissue between the superficial and deep laminae of deep fascia over the left scapulohumeral joint.

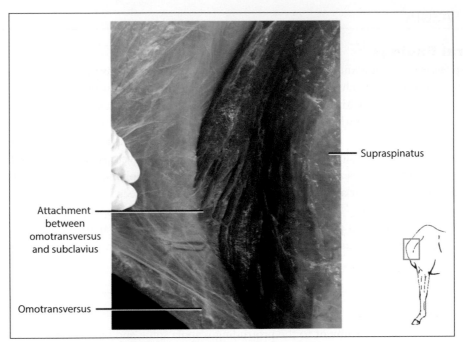

Supraspinatus

Attachment
between
omotransversus
and subclavius

Omotransversus

Fig. 5.15 Merging of the superficial lamina of deep fascia (on the underside of the omotransversus) to the epimysial fascia of the subclavius in its ventral third (left forelimb).

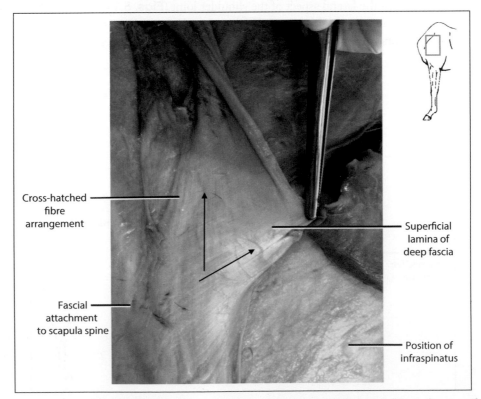

Cross-hatched
fibre
arrangement

Superficial
lamina of
deep fascia

Fascial
attachment
to scapula spine

Position of
infraspinatus

Fig. 5.16 Attachment of superficial lamina of deep fascia to the scapula spine. Note the cross hatched fibre arrangement (left forelimb).

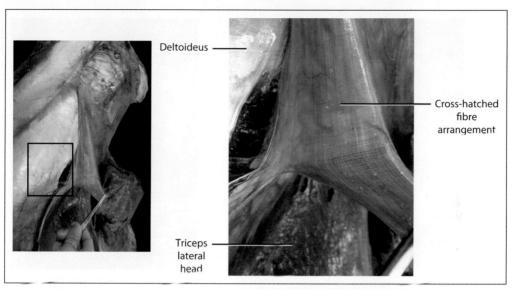

Deltoideus

Cross-hatched
fibre
arrangement

Triceps
lateral
head

Fig. 5.17 **Superficial lamina of deep fascia, caudoventral to the scapula spine. Note the cross-hatched fibre arrangement and the continuity with the muscle fibres of the deltoideus (left forelimb).**

along the margin where it joins the dorsal quarter of the deltoideus (**Fig. 5.17**). Following it cranially towards the subclavius and ventrally towards the brachiocephalicus, it thins slightly and has a parallel arrangement of fibres directed dorsoventrally. The superficial lamina does not encase the subclavius muscle but does envelop the ventral portion of the trapezius cervicis positioned superficial to its dorsal surface. Following this fascial layer down from the ventral border of trapezius cervicis, there is some variation between subjects. In some cases, the ventral border of the trapezius cervicis contacts the dorsal border of the omotransversus muscle (which is also enveloped in the superficial lamina of deep fascia). In other cases, its ventral margin is situated more dorsally and a thick expanse of fascia, with prominent dorsoventrally aligned fibres, fills the space between the two muscles (**Fig. 5.18**).

The loose connective tissue situated between the superficial lamina of deep fascia and the underlying deep lamina over these muscles is generally very loose and web-like, particularly over the scapulohumeral joint (**Figs. 5.14** and **5.19**). Over the ventral quarter of the subclavius muscle, the fascia on the underside of the brachiocephalicus – where it is continuous with the omotransversus muscle – becomes integrated with muscle fibres of the subclavius (**Fig. 5.15**) providing a point of mechanical interaction between the superficial and deep fascial laminae. Ventral to this, the superficial lamina continues from the brachiocephalicus to the medial aspect of the shoulder, forming the superficial lamina of deep fascia over the biceps brachii, coracobrachialis and TFA.

Over both the supraspinatus and infraspinatus, the superficial lamina can be easily isolated from the deep lamina encasing these muscles (**Fig. 5.20**). However, following the superficial lamina dorsocaudally from its attachment at the scapula spine, it tightly encases the trapezius thoracis. It thickens considerably on the underside of the muscle forming a smooth aponeurosis (with parallel fibres directed towards the scapula spine) which allows the muscle a relative degree of sliding over the underlying fascia of the deltoideus and the fascia associated with the scapula cartilage (**Fig. 5.21**). Extending beyond the caudal margin of this muscle it continues as a thinner sheet, much more like that over the supraspinatus, and upon reaching the latissimus dorsi, it becomes the muscle's epimysial covering.

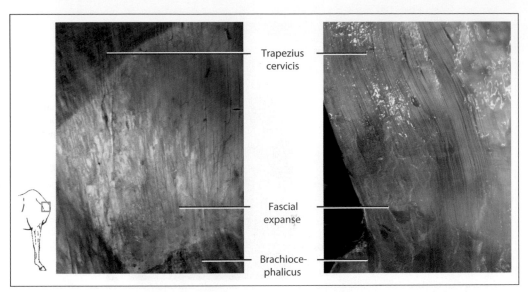

Fig. 5.18 Fascial expanse between the trapezius cervicis and omotransversus in two different subjects (left image: right forelimb; right image: left forelimb). In some cases the distal insertion of the trapezius cervicis is very close to the brachiocephalicus (right image).

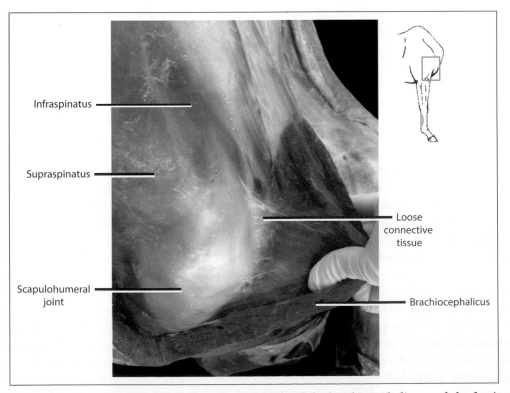

Fig. 5.19 Loose connective tissue between the underside of the brachiocephalicus and the fascia over the lateral aspect of the scapulohumeral joint (left forelimb).

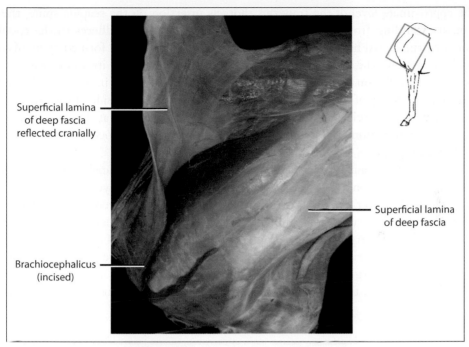

Superficial lamina
of deep fascia
reflected cranially

Superficial lamina
of deep fascia

Brachiocephalicus
(incised)

Fig. 5.20 Superficial lamina of deep fascia over the lateral aspect of the left shoulder. Fascia has been transected along the midline of the supraspinatus and through the brachiocephalicus so that it could be reflected cranially.

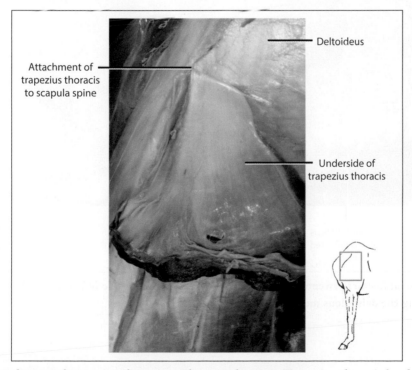

Deltoideus

Attachment of
trapezius thoracis
to scapula spine

Underside of
trapezius thoracis

Fig. 5.21 Attachment of trapezius thoracis to the scapula spine. Trapezius thoracis has been reflected ventrally to show the thickened, parallel arrangement of collagen fibres (left forelimb).

At the approximate level of the trapezius thoracis insertion on the scapula spine, the superficial lamina extending from the muscle's ventral margin strongly adheres to the aponeurotic fascia encasing the dorsal half of the deltoideus. Its caudal boundary is formed by its fusion with the deep lamina along the approximate margin of the deltoideus and its aponeurosis of origin. Additionally there is fusion of the deep and superficial laminae near the insertion of the deltoideus on the deltoid tuberosity of the humerus. Here the fascia on the underside of the brachiocephalicus integrates with the fascia encasing the deltoideus. Traction applied at this point demonstrates that it serves as a strong point of force transmission between the brachiocephalicus and deltoideus muscles (**Fig. 5.22**).

In between the trapezius thoracis and latissimus dorsi, the superficial lamina of deep fascia extends over the underlying fascia of the deltoideus as an isolated layer (**Fig. 5.21**). Over the triceps long head, however, the distinction between superficial and deep laminae is not so clear. As already described, the superficial lamina blends with the thick fascial envelope of the deltoid along the approximate margins of the deltoideus and its aponeurosis of origin. This lamina continues caudally over the triceps long head but its relationship with the muscle varies. Dorsally, and along its cranial margin (where it joins with the deltoideus) it cannot be easily separated from the muscle and can therefore be presumed to exist as (or in close relationship with) the

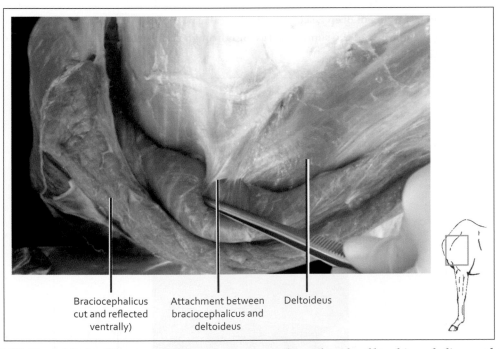

Braciocephalicus   Attachment between   Deltoideus
cut and reflected   braciocephalicus and
ventrally)   deltoideus

Fig. 5.22 Fascial fusion between the epimysial fascia on the underside of brachiocephalicus and the fascia covering the deltoideus muscle (left forelimb).

epimysial fascia of the muscle. In the mid region of the triceps long head, this fascial layer can be isolated as a thin, yet strong, membranous layer which, when followed caudally and medially, envelops the TFA.

The complexity of this layer arises slightly dorsal to the olecranon. Here it becomes continuous with the detached fascial sheet described earlier (section: superficial fascia) separating the interfascial space of the shoulder and brachium (**Fig. 5.10**). Its continuity distally is complicated by the formation of several overlapping attachments illustrated in **Fig. 5.23**. Over the cranial half of the triceps lateral head, these overlapping layers are associated with a thicker membranous layer of fascia that can be separated from the muscle and which has fibres directed caudoventrally (towards the olecranon). The positional relationship of this fascia with the muscle is maintained by fascial adhesions attaching to muscle fibres as shown in **Fig. 5.24**. Ultimately, the intramuscular connective tissue of the lateral triceps head is continuous with the superficial lamina of the deep fascia enveloping the brachiocephalicus.

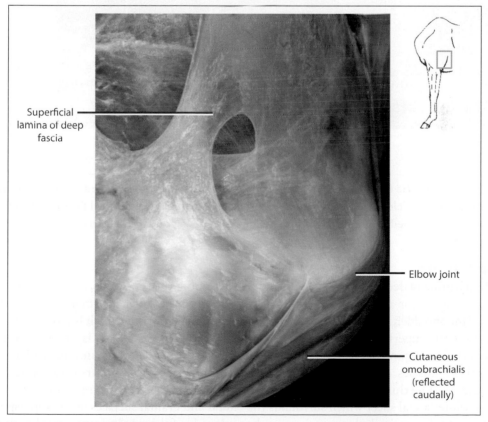

Superficial lamina of deep fascia

Elbow joint

Cutaneous omobrachialis (reflected caudally)

Fig. 5.23 Superficial lamina of deep fascia over the lateral aspect of the left brachium. Superficial fascia has been reflected caudally.

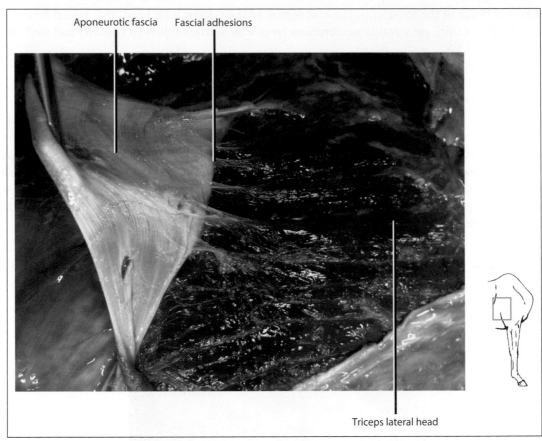

Fig. 5.24 Aponeurotic fascia of the triceps lateral head (right forelimb) reflected caudally. Fascial adhesions maintain a close connectivity between the aponeurotic and epimysial fascia of the muscle. Note also the organised arrangement of fibres comprising the aponeurotic fascia.

Deep lamina

The deep lamina of deep fascia includes the fascia enveloping the subclavius, supraspinatus, infraspinatus, teres minor and deltoideus muscles. In relation to the subclavius muscle on the cranial aspect of the shoulder, the deep fascia forms a thin epimysial covering which is loosely connected to the overlying superficial lamina described earlier. Following this fascial layer caudally, it continues as the enveloping fascia of the supraspinatus; however, no definitive intermuscular septum isolates these muscles. Instead, compartmentalisation of these muscles occurs via a change in fascial thickness. The thin fascia covering the outer surface of the subclavius transitions into a thick inelastic white fascial sheet which surrounds the lateral and cranial surfaces of the supraspinatus. In addition to this, it similarly transitions on the underside of the subclavius so that the adjoining surfaces of the two muscles have aponeurotic-like coverings that are separated by a very loose connective tissue medium (**Fig. 5.25**). Observing their connection from the medial aspect reveals strong fascial adhesions between the enveloping fasciae of the muscles.

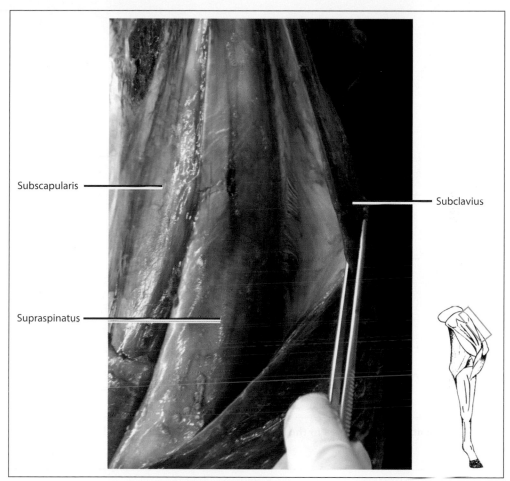

Subscapularis

Subclavius

Supraspinatus

Fig. 5.25 **Relationship between the subclavius and the dorsal half of the supraspinatus on the medial and cranial aspect of the left shoulder.**

Regarding the supraspinatus itself, the connection between the fascia and the muscle varies along its length. In the dorsal two-thirds for example, the muscle fibres insert directly onto the thick pearlescent fascia covering the muscle, thereby preventing removal of the fascia (**Fig. 5.26**). In contrast, the fascia extending from the subclavius over the ventral half of the supraspinatus can be easily removed due to the formation of an additional deep layer (**Fig. 5.27**). Both of these layers continue ventrally over the scapulohumeral joint. The thinner deeper layer merges with the fascia comprising the shoulder joint capsule and with the insertion of the supraspinatus and infraspinatus. It cannot be isolated from the supraspinatus without disrupting the integrity of the muscle. In relation to the infraspinatus muscle, fascial reinforcements which integrate with its tendon of insertion are present. These are directed

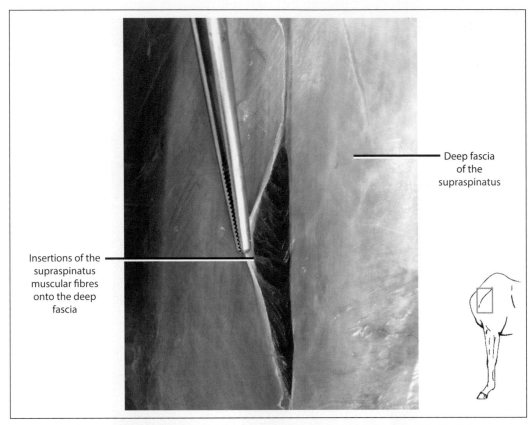

Deep fascia of the supraspinatus

Insertions of the supraspinatus muscular fibres onto the deep fascia

Fig. 5.26 **Attachment of muscle fibres to the aponeurotic fascia over the dorsal half of the supraspinatus.**

The relationship between fascial force transmission and muscular contractions comes down to the connectivity between fascia and muscle fibers. Stecco et al. (2009b) proposed that transmission of forces by fascia potentially creates a stretch which is translated into muscle spindles in the epimysium or endomysium. This could allow muscular contractions to be modulated by "peripheral demands" thereby presenting an anatomical basis for peripheral motor control. This idea suggests that the interaction between muscles and their fascial covering largely influences their functionality and autonomy. A close connection between fascia and muscles would enable a two-way interaction through which the fascia either takes on the contraction state of its enveloped muscle, or the contraction state of the muscle is influenced or initiated by the tensional forces transmitted through the fascia. Similar to observations made on the human pectoralis major muscle (Stecco et al. 2009a), a true epimysium was not identified for several muscles in the brachium and shoulder, particularly over the lateral aspect of the scapula (supraspinatus, infraspinatus and deltoideus). Histological investigations in the human pectoralis major revealed that, in such cases, the deep aponeurotic fascia takes on the role of an epimysium and it was further concluded that this type of relationship allows selective spatial stretching of fascia and zonal muscle activation (Stecco et al. 2009b). Whilst the structure of the deep fascia may indicate a role reflective of an epimysium, observations from this present study do not give credence to the idea of selective spatial stretching or zonal muscle activation. Indeed, several muscles in this study inserted directly into their surrounding fascia.

However, selective functioning of these muscles seems unlikely due to the continuity of fascia across them. For example, traction applied to the deep fascia on the lateral aspect of the scapulohumeral joint was clearly observed to transmit across to the supraspinatus, infraspinatus, deltoideus and triceps, strongly suggesting that the deep fascia over the lateral aspect of the shoulder joint does not allow functional autonomy of the associated muscles. This makes redundant the classical anatomy technique and viewpoint of isolating muscles and considering their function in terms of their points of origin and insertion.

In addition to this, it introduces a new concept to consider in exercising horses. Recent research has demonstrated how a substantial amount of stress generated through active contractility of the muscle is transmitted to the fascia during exercise (Findley, Chaudhry, & Dhar 2015). This present study shows that externally applied forces are similarly transmitted and redistributed through the fascia and its muscular attachments. Hence, in terms of riding and extensive training for various performance disciplines, this idea strongly suggests that exercise therapies and methods of rehabilitation need to be tailored to manage fascial as well as muscular stress.

In addition to this, the continuity of the fascia over the shoulder region may also be part of the reason why the pectoral girdle is rarely subject to overuse injury (MacDonald, Kannegieter, Peroni, & Merfy 2006). It allows for an even distribution of forces so that no one muscle or attachment point is overloaded. It also allows for coordination between muscles and bones (for example, the attachment to the scapula spine and lateral humeral shaft), whilst reducing the neural input required. This is a particularly important aspect of equine locomotion during fast exercise as there may not be time for neural feedback and stimulation of muscles through complex neural pathways.

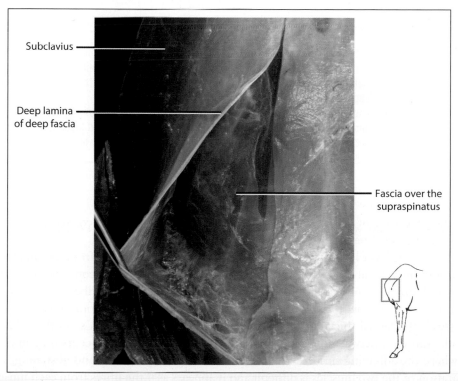

Fig. 5.27 Deep lamina of deep fascia over the distal half of the supraspinatus. Note how, ventrally, the deep lamina is connected with loose connective tissue to a secondary layer over the supraspinatus. Dorsally, these layers join and become integrated with the epimysial fascia of the muscle (left forelimb).

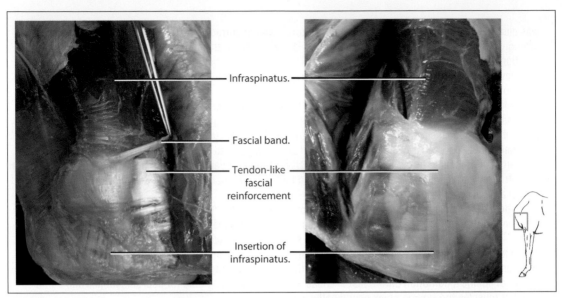

Infraspinatus.

Fascial band.

Tendon-like
fascial
reinforcement

Insertion of
infraspinatus.

Fig. 5.28 Fascial bands integrating with the insertion of infraspinatus. Each of these continues cau-dally and remains superficial to the teres minor. They are inseparable from the tendon of insertion of the infraspinatus (left forelimb).

Ligaments of the shoulder joint

According to Nickel et al. (1986), there are no distinct ligaments associated with the shoulder joint and the stability of the joint is instead maintained via the insertion of shoulder and brachial muscles. Here, we see an additional fascial reinforcement which may contribute to joint stability. It is observed in close association with the infraspinatus tendon of insertion.

The definitive margins and thickness of this reinforced band was inconsistent among subjects supporting the idea that fascial architecture is dependent on individual loading and locomotory patterns. Such differences may be reflected in the stability and locomotory efficiency of the limb.

towards the insertion of the deltoideus and teres minor and have inconsistent margins and thickness among specimens (**Fig. 5.28**).

The aponeurotic layer lying superficial to this (and extending caudally from the subclavius mus-cle) forms a strong fascial sheet over the scapulohumeral joint and also continues over the infra-spinatus and deltoideus muscles (**Fig. 5.29**). Similar to the situation described earlier, there are no distinct intermuscular septa formed between these muscles despite the continuity of fascia across them. Instead, the fascial thickness and connection varies to allow for a smooth gliding surface between the muscles. Between the supraspinatus and infraspinatus, this occurs only in the ventral quarter where the adjoining surfaces are both characteristically smooth and glistening. Dorsal to this, separation of the two muscles is difficult and it appears as if the fibres from each muscle insert on either side of a single fascial sheet dividing the two.

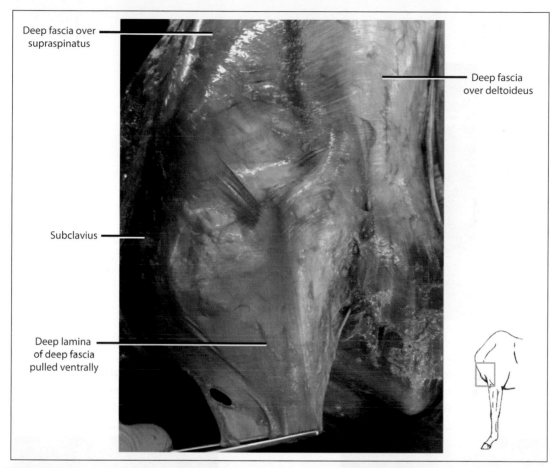

Deep fascia over suprspinatus

Deep fascia over deltoideus

Subclavius

Deep lamina of deep fascia pulled ventrally

Fig. 5.29 Deep lamina of deep fascia over the lateral aspect of the left scapulohumeral joint. Note the parallel fibre arrangement and its continuity over the supraspinatus, infraspinatus and deltoideus dorsally.

The relationship between the infraspinatus and deltoideus is slightly different. The underside of deltoideus which rests upon the ventral third of the infraspinatus is thick, smooth and has a white pearlescent appearance (**Fig. 5.30**). It is mostly unattached to the epimysial fascia of the ventral end of the infraspinatus (and the small area of teres minor situated immediately caudal to it), but does merge along its caudal margin to create a closed space (**Fig. 5.30**). In the mid region of the scapula, fascial adhesions are present between the infraspinatus and underside of the deltoideus so that the deltoideus cannot be removed without disrupting the integrity of the underlying infraspinatus muscle (**Fig. 5.31**). The fascia over the lateral surface of the deltoideus itself is similar to that over the dorsal half of the supraspinatus. It integrates with the muscle's endomysium and provides an insertion for individual muscle fibres (**Fig. 5.32**). On its underside, it fuses with the fascia of the triceps long head so that an impenetrable boundary is formed (**Fig. 5.30**).

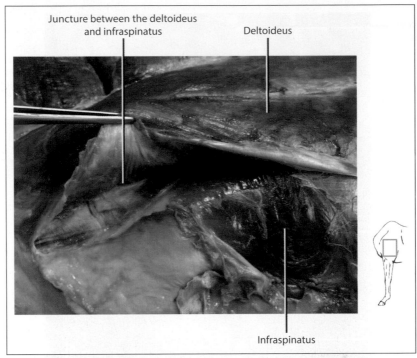

Fig. 5.30 Fusion between fascia of the deltoideus and infraspinatus, forming a closed fascial boundary. Fascia extending across the ventral extremity of the infraspinatus from the deltoideus has been severed to show the relationship between the muscles where they sit against each other (left forelimb).

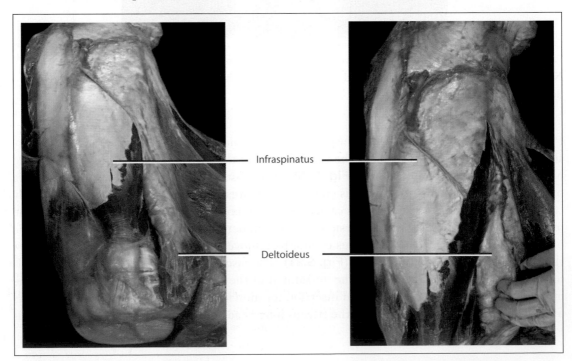

Fig. 5.31 Relationship between the infraspinatus and the enveloping fascia of the deltoideus (left forelimb).

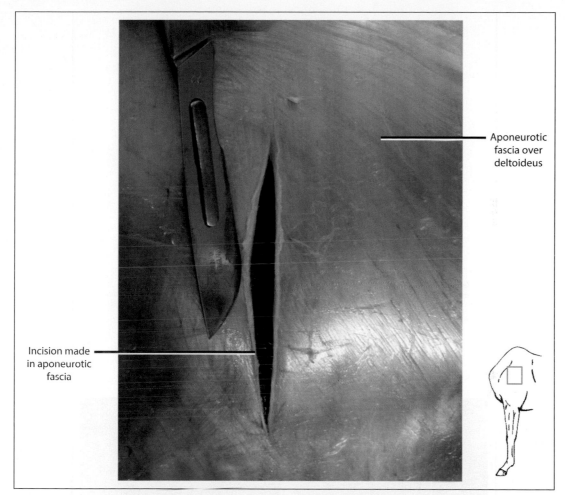

Aponeurotic
fascia over
deltoideus

Incision made
in aponeurotic
fascia

Fig. 5.32 Incision made in the aponeurotic fascia of the deltoideus (at the approximate level of the scapula spine). Note its thickness and its integration with the fibres comprising the muscle.

In reference to the triceps muscle and teres minor, the fascia covering the underside of the deltoideus which overlies these muscles is much thinner and more transparent than the rest of the muscle's fascial covering. The smooth gliding surface between the adjoining surfaces is achieved through thickening of the triceps and teres minor fascia. **Figs. 5.33** and **5.34** show how the thickened fascia over these muscles has fibres directed caudoventrally and, from the underside of deltoideus, it joins along the muscles cranial border to form a closed, impenetrable boundary. Dorsally, the fascia enveloping the long head of the triceps blends with the scapula cartilage.

A similar attachment is present between the triceps lateral head and the deltoideus. In this case, the triceps lateral head has a thin epimysial fascial covering which moves easily against the aponeurotic covering of the deltoideus. Cranioventrally, the thick fascia covering the triceps lateral head described earlier continues over the extensor carpi radialis and biceps brachii. It also has strong attachments to the lateral surface of the humeral shaft (**Figs. 5.35** and **5.36**).

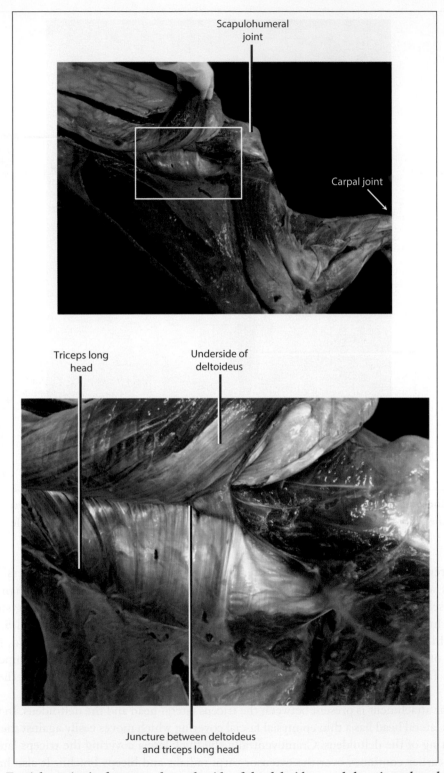

Fig. 5.33 Fascial continuity between the underside of the deltoideus and the triceps long head (right forelimb)- lateral aspect.

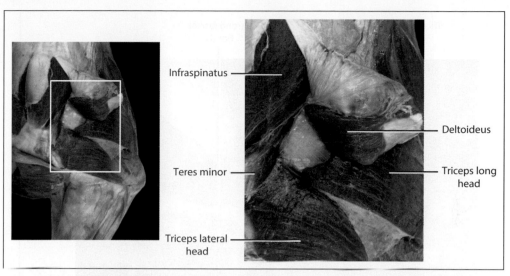

Fig. 5.34 Change in fascial thickness over the deltoideus and the lateral and long heads of the triceps (cranial aspect of left forelimb).

Post-anaesthetic myopathy

The most clinically relevant fascial compartment observed was that formed between the long head of the triceps and the deltoideus on the lateral aspect, and the long head of the triceps and both the latissimus dorsi and teres major on the medial aspect. The impenetrable boundary formed by the fusion of fascia from these muscles creates an enclosed space in which fluid can accumulate without being redistributed as would occur with limb movement and muscular contraction. This helps to explain why the triceps (and sometimes the flexor muscles of the antebrachium) are one of the most commonly affected muscles with respect to post-anaesthetic myopathy (Kobluk, 1995; Norman, Williams, Dodman, & Kraus 1989).

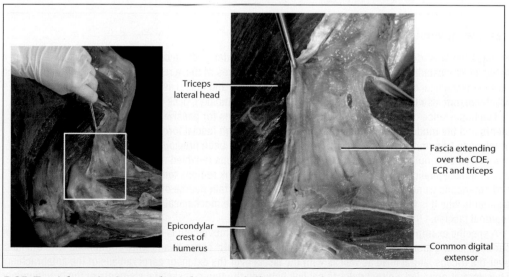

Fig. 5.35 Fascial continuity over lateral aspect of elbow joint where the extensor carpi radialis and triceps lateral head meet. The fascia here has a strong attachment to the epicondylar crest of the humerus (right forelimb).

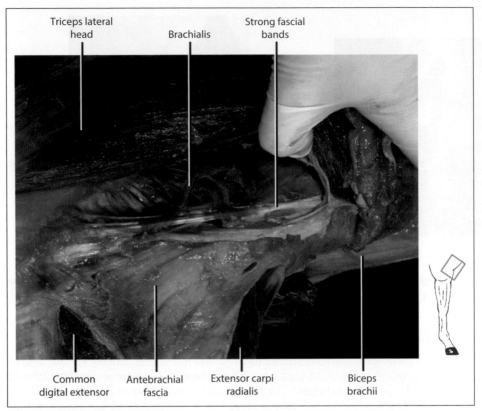

Triceps lateral head   Brachialis   Strong fascial bands

Common digital extensor   Antebrachial fascia   Extensor carpi radialis   Biceps brachii

Fig. 5.36 Continuity between deep fascia of the brachium and deep fascia of the antebrachium. Note the attachment of the antebrachial fascia to the epicondylar crest of the humerus and the continuity of this fascia with that over the biceps brachii proximal to the reinforced fascial bands (right forelimb).

Passive movement

Perhaps the most distinguishing characteristic of the shoulder girdle and brachial fascia was its continuity between all musculoskeletal, vascular and nervous structures of these regions. This allowed for an uninterrupted mechanical connection between not only the medial and lateral aspects of the shoulder girdle and brachium, but also between these regions and the trunk (caudally), neck (cranially) and forearm (distally).

The importance of this connectivity lies in its implications for passive movement between limb segments and the modulation of muscular contractions through fascial force transmission. The capacity of fascia to transmit tensional forces across segments has been previously demonstrated. Hence, the myofascial continuity between the shoulder and neck regions (enabled mostly through the pectorals and brachiocephalicus), and between the shoulder and trunk regions (enabled through latissimus dorsi and cutaneous trunci) strongly suggests that there is a certain degree of coordination between these segments which is facilitated throughout locomotion by the mechanical connectivity of the respective regional fasciae.

A specific example of this potentially passively-enabled movement is demonstrated through the fascial bands inserting along the lateral aspect of the humeral shaft. These bands were continuous with the fascia over the triceps lateral head as well as with the fascia over the extensor carpi radialis of the antebrachium. Therefore, it provided a direct mechanical link between the musculoskeletal elements of the brachium and antebrachium which likely serves to facilitate elbow joint movement.

MEDIAL ASPECT

The fascia over the medial aspect of the shoulder and brachium is complex and difficult to discern due to the presence of the axillary vessels and nerves. No distinct superficial layer is clear; however, similar to the lateral aspect, there are two separate laminae of deep fascia which are interconnected at several points.

Superficial lamina

The superficial lamina is most easily identified by its continuation with the subclavius in the dorsal half of the shoulder region, and by its continuation with the pectoralis ascendens, pectoralis transversus and brachiocephalicus in the ventral half of the shoulder region. In this way, the superficial lamina of the medial aspect is an extension of both the superficial and deep laminae described over the lateral aspect of the brachium and shoulder.

In the ventral half of the shoulder region, superficial to the aponeurotic extension of the latissimus dorsi, the superficial lamina provides the insertion for the cutaneous trunci muscle, which takes the form of a reinforced fascial band tapering on approach to the scapulohumeral joint (**Fig. 5.37**). Cranially, it becomes continuous with the fascia enveloping the superficial and deep

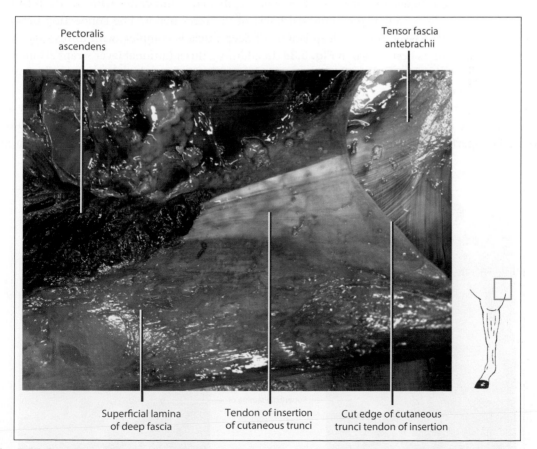

Fig. 5.37 **Insertion of cutaneous trunci into the axillary fascia. Note the continuity it has with pectoralis ascendens and the fascia, which extends ventrally over the TFA. Only the most cranial portion of this tendon is visible. The remaining caudal part was severed (medial aspect of right forelimb).**

pectoral muscles (as well as the brachiocephalicus), whilst ventrally, it continues as a thin sheet which spreads over the TFA, biceps brachii and coracobrachialis. Through its association with the ascending pectoral, it additionally has a strong point of connection to the deep fascia. This connection occurs near the point of insertion of the pectoralis ascendens muscle on the lateral epicondyle of the humerus and the tendon of origin of the coracobrachialis muscle.

Dorsal to the cutaneous trunci fascial band, the superficial lamina continues as the epimysial fascia surrounding the teres major muscle. As it does so, it encases the lateral thoracic vein as well as the dorsal thoracic vein and artery. Over the dorsal two-thirds of the teres major muscle, the superficial lamina thickens to form a white pearlescent covering which becomes continuous with the aponeurotic fascia of the subscapularis (discussed further in the following). In addition to this, it also transitions into the epimysial fascia of the latissimus dorsi caudally.

In relation to the subscapularis, a superficial lamina can often be isolated. It exists as an extension of the fascia enveloping the pectoralis ascendens and subclavius. It should also be noted that as this fascia courses dorsally from the pectoralis ascendens, it integrates with the axillary arteries, veins and nerves emerging from that area. The superficial lamina of fascia over the subscapularis is thickest at the most ventral and cranial margins of the muscle. Here, it gives rise to an additional deep layer on its deep surface which blends with the deep lamina in the mid region of the muscle. Along the caudoventral margin of the muscle, this layer integrates with the deep lamina covering the muscle as well as the epimysial fascia of the teres major. The connection between this additional fascial layer and the deep lamina of deep fascia is complex, with fibres varying in their direction. This is best shown in **Fig. 5.38**. In addition, this additional layer wraps around the cranial surface of the subscapularis in its ventral half to isolate it from the adjoining surface of the supraspinatus muscle.

Over the dorsal margin of the subscapularis, the main superficial lamina attaches strongly and abruptly to the deep lamina along the serrated margins of the scapula (**Fig. 5.39**). Dorsal to this point, the superficial lamina integrates with the serratus ventralis cervicis. Along the ventral margin

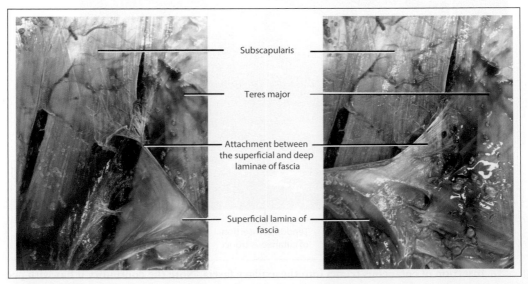

Subscapularis

Teres major

Attachment between the superficial and deep laminae of fascia

Superficial lamina of fascia

Fig. 5.38 Fascial continuity between the subscapularis and teres major over the medial aspect of the right shoulder.

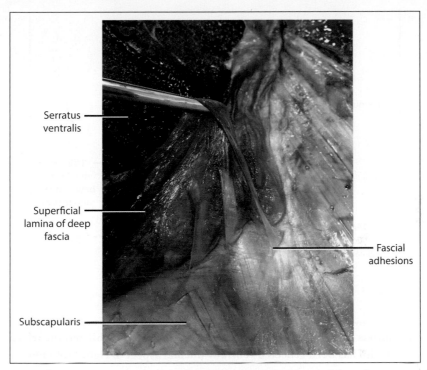

Serratus ventralis

Superficial lamina of deep fascia

Fascial adhesions

Subscapularis

Fig. 5.39 Fascial adhesions between the superficial and deep laminae of deep fascia over the proximal quarter of the subscapularis (medial aspect of right forelimb).

of this muscle, the superficial lamina thickens as it continues caudally and displays a tendon-like appearance with fibres directed caudodistally. The continuation of this may be an extension of the serratus ventralis thoracis.

Deep lamina

In the ventral half of the scapula region, the deep lamina of deep fascia can be followed most easily from the latissimus dorsi and its aponeurotic extension. Here, the deep lamina (which integrated with the latissimus dorsi) continues ventrally as the epimysial fascia of the TFA. Hence, through the insertion of the TFA into the antebrachial fascia, a direct continuation between the trunk (via the latissimus dorsi), brachium and antebrachium is formed.

Along the caudal and cranial margins of the TFA, the deep lamina transitions into the epimysial fascia of the triceps long head. For the most part, loose connective tissue separates the deep surfaces of these muscles to allow for a friction reduced space. However, immediately dorsal to the olecranon, an inelastic and fibrous area strongly connects the two muscles (**Fig. 5.40**). By following the TFA and triceps cranially, the deep lamina appears to form fascial sheaths around the brachial vessels and nerve before continuing across to form a thick fascial expanse over the biceps brachii and coracobrachialis (**Fig. 5.41**). For the most part, the fascia over the coracobrachialis and biceps brachii can be readily isolated from the muscles; however, at the most craniodorsal point of the coracobrachialis, it adheres on its superficial surface to the superficial lamina enveloping the pectoralis ascendens (**Fig. 5.42**). Thick fascial reinforcement have been observed in this fascia crossing from the biceps to the attachment between the coracobrachialis and the pectoralis ascendens (**Fig. 5.43**). Between the

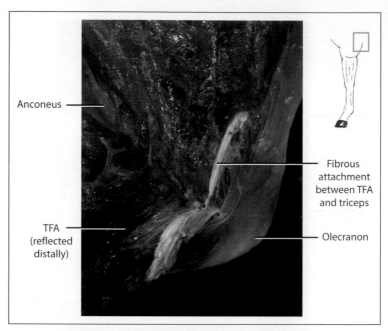

Anconeus

Fibrous attachment between TFA and triceps

TFA (reflected distally)

Olecranon

Fig. 5.40 Strong fibrous attachment between the tensor fascia antebrachii and the triceps. The tensor fascia antebrachii has been reflected ventrally (medial aspect of right forelimb).

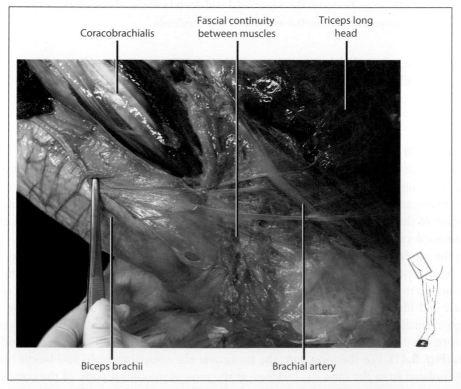

Coracobrachialis

Fascial continuity between muscles

Triceps long head

Biceps brachii

Brachial artery

Fig. 5.41 Extension of fascia from the triceps to the biceps brachii and coracobrachialis (TFA has been removed). This fascia compartmentalises the coracobrachialis and biceps brachii. Note how the brachial artery is encased within this fascia also (medial aspect of right forelimb).

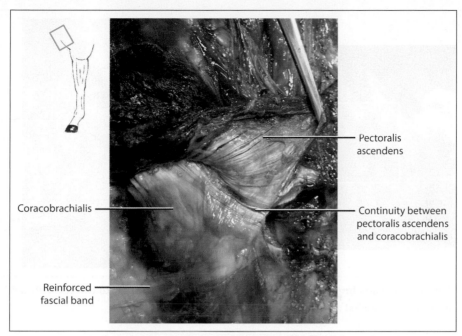

Pectoralis
ascendens

Coracobrachialis

Continuity between
pectoralis ascendens
and coracobrachialis

Reinforced
fascial band

Fig. 5.42 Continuity between the ascending pectorals and the coracobrachialis in the right forelimb (medial aspect). The reinforced fascial band was not present in all specimens, but it is shown here as a prominent band connecting the coracobrachialis, biceps brachii (ventral to it) and the tensor fascia antebrachii (caudal to it).

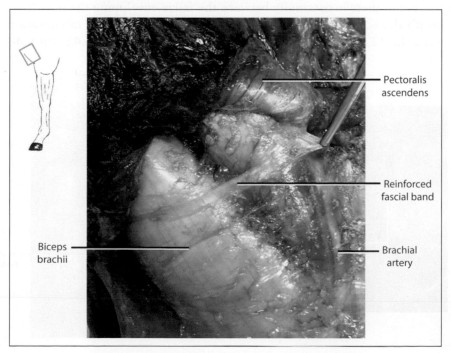

Pectoralis
ascendens

Reinforced
fascial band

Biceps
brachii

Brachial
artery

Fig. 5.43 Fascial reinforcement in deep fascia over biceps brachii and coracobrachialis (medial aspect of right forelimb).

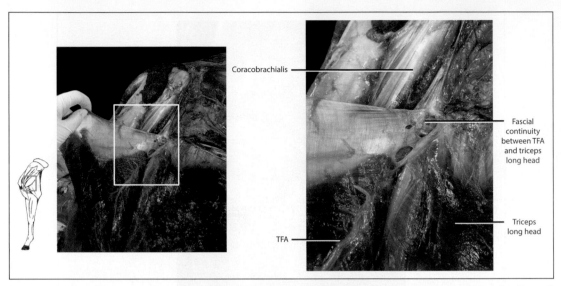

Fig. 5.44 **Tensor fascia antebrachii reflected cranially and its attachment to the coracobrachialis and the underlying triceps (medial aspect of right forelimb).**

coracobrachialis and the biceps brachii, the deep fascia extending from the TFA gives rise to a distinct intermuscular septum which is traversed by branches of the brachial artery. Over the ventral surface of the biceps brachii it continues as the fascia of the pectoralis descendens and brachiocephalicus.

A notable point of stronger connectivity exists between the coracobrachialis and the TFA where the fascia envelops the brachial vessels and nerves. This is illustrated in **Fig. 5.44**. Through this point, there is continuity between the fascia enveloping the muscles of the ventral and dorsal halves of the shoulder region. There is a more complex organisation of fascial layers between the TFA and ventral half of the biceps brachii. **Figs. 5.45** and **5.46** illustrate

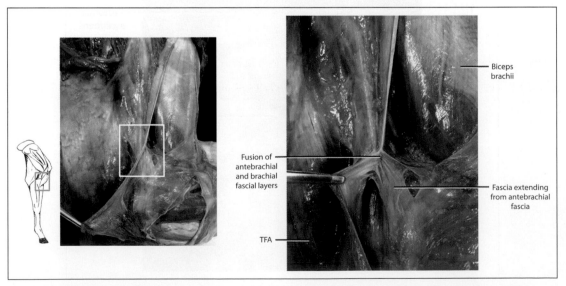

Fig. 5.45 **Attachment of fascial layers derived from the tensor fascia antebrachii over the medial aspect of the left brachium.**

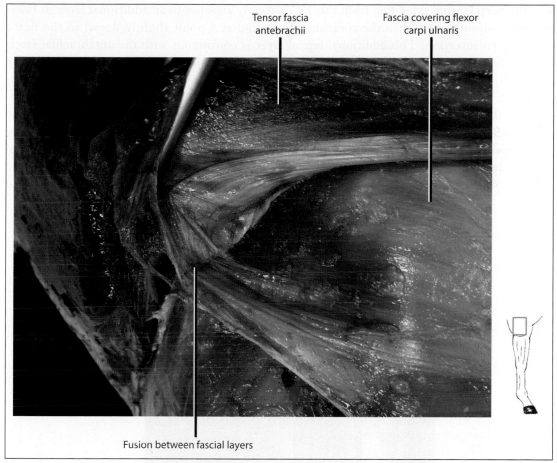

Tensor fascia
antebrachii

Fascia covering flexor
carpi ulnaris

Fusion between fascial layers

Fig. 5.46 Fusion between fascial layers over the medial aspect of the brachium and antebrachium
(left forelimb).

Vessels and nerves

Fascial sheaths surrounding the brachial plexus and associated vascular structures at the ventral end of
the subscapularis were very much derived from the deep and superficial laminae of the axillary fascia. It
has already been discussed how a substantial amount of force generated by muscle activity is transmitted through the connected fascia. Hence, based on earlier studies demonstrating how fascial tension
increases venous pressure and helps with venous blood return (Garfin et al., 1981), it is likely that blood
flow throughout the equine shoulder and distal limb is facilitated by the contractility of the surrounding
muscles and their enveloping fascia.

how the deep lamina extending from the TFA strongly attaches to an additional layer of fascia at a point slightly ventral to the coracobrachialis and at a point slightly dorsal to the flexor carpi ulnaris insertion. This additional fascial layer is continuous with the antebrachial fascia over the flexor carpi radialis and flexor carpi ulnaris. It is easily separable from the underlying and overlying tissues, and it has strong directional fibres which cross the proximal extremity of the flexor carpi radialis horizontally and the ventral end of the biceps brachii diagonally. In the mid region of the biceps brachii it blends with the muscle's epimysial covering (**Fig. 5.45**). Cutting through these connections and reflecting the TFA dorsocaudally more clearly reveals the relationship between the brachial vessels and nerves and the deep lamina of deep fascia, demonstrating how the vessels traverse the fascia rather than being encased within it (**Fig. 5.47**). They are additionally closely bound to the coracobrachialis by the muscle's own

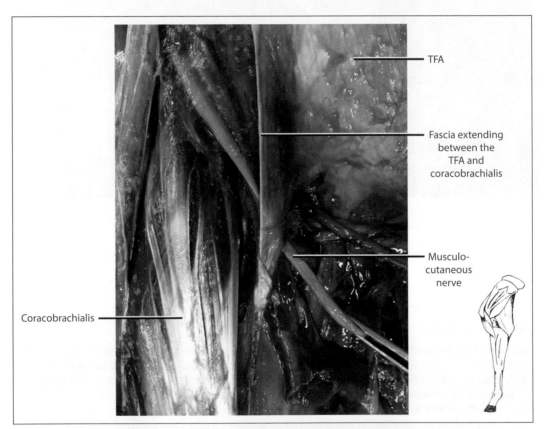

Fig. 5.47 Fascial continuity between the tensor fascia antebrachii and coracobrachialis. Note the relationship of the musculocutaneous nerve (right forelimb).

epimysial fascia, which extends across to the deep surface of the triceps medial and long heads. Traction applied at the point of attachment between the deep lamina and this additional layer shows a prominent line of tension distribution into the coracobrachialis and biceps brachii and even into the proximal antebrachium (cranial aspect) where the lacertus fibrosus is situated (**Video 7.1, clips 4–5**).

Following the fascia from the dorsal margin of the TFA, it continues and thickens to form the aponeurotic fascial insertion of the latissimus dorsi. The fibres comprising this fascial expanse form a white glistening surface and are oriented parallel to each other in a cranioventral direction (**Fig. 5.48**). Hence there is very limited stretch possible in that direction, and only a slight degree more in the caudoventral direction. On the underside of this aponeurosis, very strong directional attachments to the epimysial fascia of the medial surface of triceps long head are present. These attachments are illustrated in **Figs. 5.49** and **5.50**. Additionally there are attachments between the triceps long head and teres major (**Fig. 5.51**). The strength of these attachments is reinforced by a thickening of the triceps fascia. **Figs. 5.52–5.54** illustrate a gradually more defined orientation of fibres with a pearlescent appearance in the dorsal half of the triceps long head (medial surface). Dorsocranially, these fibres form thick strands (**Fig. 5.55**) and merge with the fascia of the latissimus dorsi to form an enclosed space that is separated from the teres major and subscapularis.

Investigation of the relationship between teres major and the latissimus dorsi demonstrates close physical connectivity between the two muscles, similar to that between the subscapularis and supraspinatus. The underside of the teres major directly attaches to the aponeurosis of the latissimus dorsi (**Fig. 5.48**). Dorsal to this, the adjoining surfaces of the two muscle bellies are not separated via an intermuscular septum. Rather, loose connective tissue provides enough of a barrier to maintain the muscles as two separate entities without affording much movement between them. Through this continuity with the teres major, the latissimus dorsi attaches to the teres tubercle (**Fig. 5.56**) and becomes continuous with the subscapularis.

The subscapularis is enveloped by an aponeurotic fascial layer with mostly dorsoventrally directed fibres (**Fig. 5.57**) but some fibres of varying orientation also exist (**Fig. 5.58**). These fibres give a fading iridescent appearance in the ventral direction. The attachment of this fascia to the muscle fibres varies among individuals. In some cases, it can be cleanly removed from the muscle surface over from its ventral margin to the line of attachment described earlier for the superficial lamina. In other cases, it cannot be removed without disrupting the integrity of the muscle. When it can be removed, several of the small subscapular nerves are clearly evident. Ventrally, it continues with the deep fascia of the coracobrachialis and, by extension, the biceps brachii and TFA as well. Along its ventral margin, a reinforced fascial band is observed which originates from the fascia of the teres major, and continues as a horizontal band over the cranial surface of the subclavius (**Fig. 5.59**). This fascia is intricately arranged around the axillary artery, vein and nerve. Along its cranial surface, the subscapularis is separated via loose connective tissue to the adjoining surface of the supraspinatus.

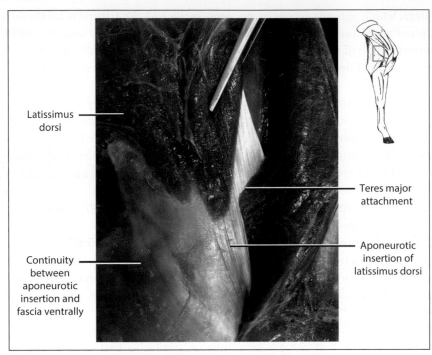

Latissimus dorsi

Teres major attachment

Aponeurotic insertion of latissimus dorsi

Continuity between aponeurotic insertion and fascia ventrally

Fig. 5.48 Aponeurotic extension of the latissimus dorsi. Note the attachment of the teres major and its continuity with the fascia extending over the tensor fascia antebrachii ventrally (medial aspect of left forelimb).

The latissimus dorsi and cutaneous trunci

The latissimus dorsi and the cutaneous trunci both have their main muscle bellies situated in the trunk region, superficial to the thoracic cage. The latissimus dorsi arises from the supraspinous ligaments and from the thoracolumbar fascia (Nickel et al., 1986) and inserts on the medial aspect of the teres tubercle with the TFA and teres major (Dyce et al., 2002; Nickel et al., 1986; Sisson & Grossman, 1938). According to Nickel et al. (1986), this tendon of insertion is relatively weak. Investigation of the fascia in this area demonstrates this weakness to be compensated for by the connectivity of its preceding aponeurosis which became continuous ventrally with the epimysial fascia of the TFA and strongly attached to the deep epimysial surface of the teres major. It has been suggested that the insertion of muscles via aponeurotic sheets is optimal for high speed contraction over a wide range of motion but at the expense of force development (Payne, Veenman, & Wilson 2005). This appears to be the case in relation to the aponeurosis of the latissimus dorsi. The latissimus dorsi is a primary limb retractor (Payne et al., 2005) and hence high speed retraction over a wide range of motion is paramount. The compromise of this (decreased force development) is likely compensated for through the connectivity it has to the teres major and the TFA. Muscles can distribute a significant part of their contractile forces onto fascial structures (Findley 2012). In the case of the latissimus dorsi, its aponeurotic extension is continuous with the teres major and TFA and hence its function may in fact be mediated by the simultaneous activity of these muscles (which function to flex the shoulder and extend the elbow joint [Sisson & Grossman, 1938]). This suggests that the fascial continuity between these muscles serves as both a passive coordinating mechanism and a medium through which active muscle contractility is stimulated.

The cutaneous trunci on the other hand is a superficial muscle responsible for the skin-twitch reflex which occurs in response to tactile stimulation over the lateral trunk region (Essig et al., 2013). The possibility of the cutaneous trunci having a more prominent locomotory function has not previously been discussed, most likely due to the superficial positioning of the muscle and its relative muscle mass (as demonstrated by van Iwaarden , Stubbs, & Clayton (2012)). However, in considering this muscle from a mechanically-integrated perspective, the insertions of the cutaneous trunci muscle suggest that the muscle may, to a small degree, facilitate forelimb retraction. In this present study, the cutaneous trunci was described to be continuous with the fascia enveloping the superficial and deep pectorals (and, by extension, the brachiocephalicus) as well as with the TFA and the triceps long and lateral heads. This supports previous findings which have described the cutaneous trunci to have tendinous connections to the teres major (van Iwaarden et al., 2012) and pectoral fascia (Nickel et al., 1986). To the authors' knowledge, no discussion has yet been put forth regarding the potential functional significance of these connections. The pectoralis profundus has a role in retracting the limb (Sisson & Grossman, 1938) as it is active throughout the early swing phase and throughout most of the stance phase (Preedy [1998], cited by Payne et al. [2005]).The triceps and TFA on the other hand, are both involved in extension of the elbow (Sisson & Grossman, 1938). Elbow extension increases throughout the stance phase and reaches maximum extension at the end of the stance phase (Back et al., 1995) indicating that the triceps and TFA both contribute to retraction of the limb when it is under load. The extensive connectivity of these muscles and the pectoralis profundus with the cutaneous trunci further suggests that it too may contribute, through passive mechanical means, to forelimb retraction throughout locomotion. Additionally, further investigations into how it relates to the thoracolumbar fascia and the fascia of the proximal hindlimb may elucidate mechanical connectivity which contributes to the coordination of the fore- and hindlimbs.

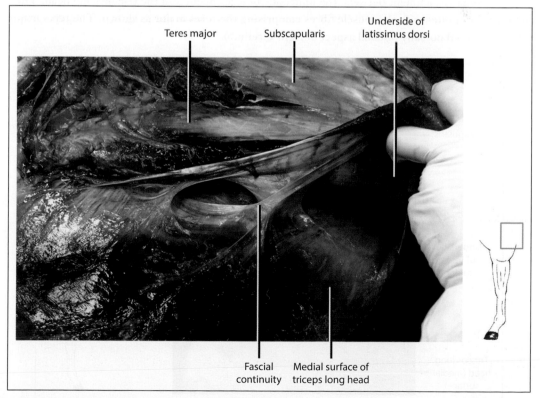

Fig. 5.49 Complex connectivity between fascia of the latissimus dorsi, teres major and the underside of the triceps long head (medial aspect of right forelimb).

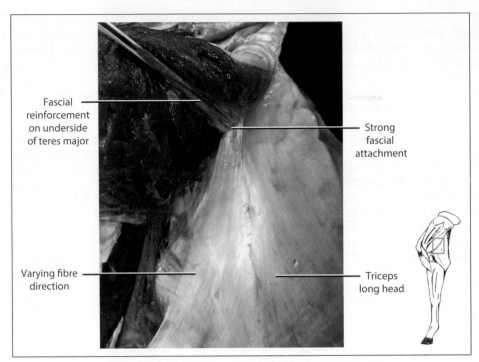

Fig. 5.50 Fascial attachment between the underside of teres major and the triceps long head. This attachment integrates with the muscle fibres comprising the teres major as shown. The teres major has been reflected dorsally (medial aspect of right forelimb).

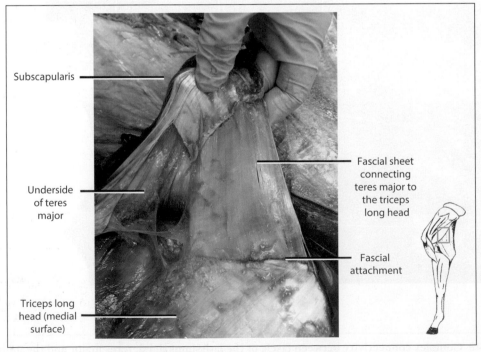

Fig. 5.51 Fascial sheet connecting the aponeurosis of latissimus dorsi to the fascia of the triceps long head (medial aspect of right forelimb).

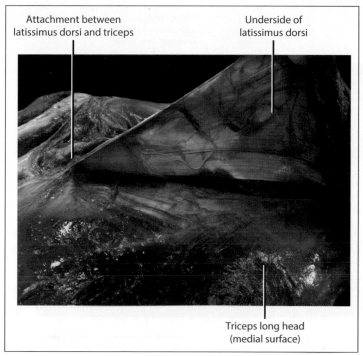

Fig. 5.52 Fusion between aponeurotic insertion of the latissimus dorsi and the epimysial fascia of the triceps long head. Attachments illustrated in Fig. 5.49 have been severed (medial aspect of right forelimb).

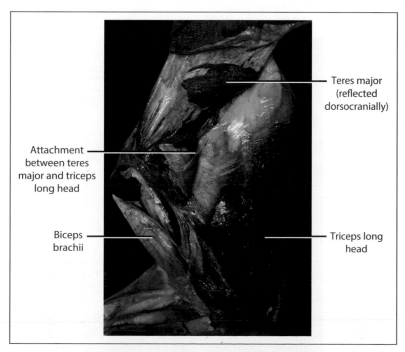

Fig. 5.53 Change in fascial thickness over medial aspect of the triceps lateral head. The tensor fascia antebrachii has been removed and the teres major has been reflected dorsocranially (medial aspect of right forelimb).

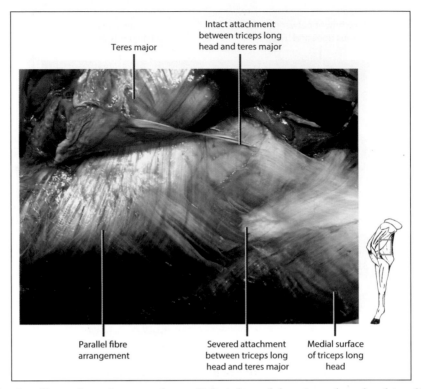

Teres major

Intact attachment
between triceps long
head and teres major

Parallel fibre
arrangement

Severed attachment
between triceps long
head and teres major

Medial surface
of triceps long
head

Fig. 5.54 Varying fibre orientation over the medial surface of the triceps long head (medial aspect of right forelimb).

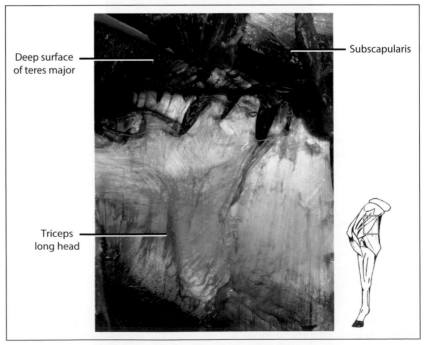

Deep surface
of teres major

Subscapularis

Triceps
long head

Fig. 5.55 Fascia over the medial aspect of the triceps long head at its most dorsocranial margin. The latissimus dorsi and teres major have been reflected dorsally (medial aspect of right forelimb).

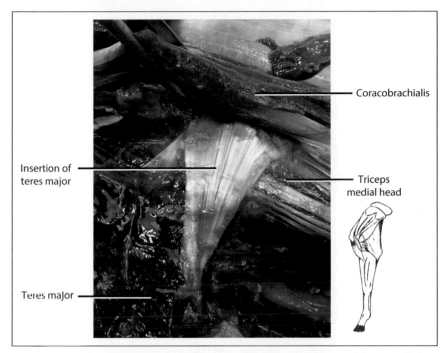

Coracobrachialis

Insertion of
teres major

Triceps
medial head

Teres major

Fig. 5.56 Conjoined tendon of insertion of the teres major and latissimus dorsi (medial aspect of right forelimb).

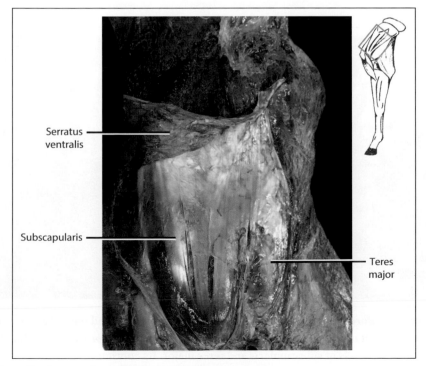

Serratus
ventralis

Subscapularis

Teres
major

Fig. 5.57 Deep fascia over the subscapularis (right forelimb).

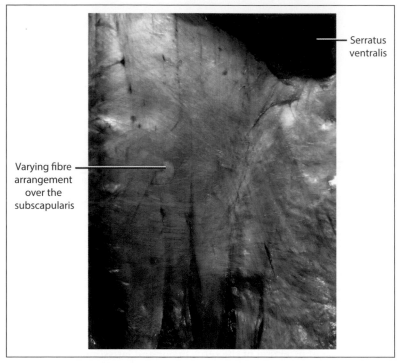

Serratus ventralis

Varying fibre arrangement over the subscapularis

Fig. 5.58 Varying orientation of fibres comprising the aponeurotic fascia of the subscapularis (right forelimb).

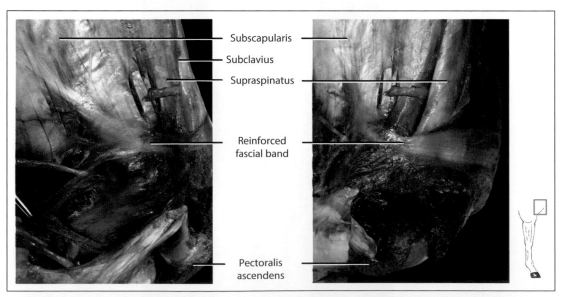

Subscapularis

Subclavius

Supraspinatus

Reinforced fascial band

Pectoralis ascendens

Fig. 5.59 Fascial reinforcements connecting muscles over the cranial and medial aspects of the left shoulder. The proximal reinforced fascial band continues around the supraspinatus; the distal band extends over the distal ends of subscapularis and teres major. Its continuity with the vessels and nerves of this area has been cut away for clarity.

REFERENCES

Back, W., Schamhardt, H., Savelberg, H., van den Bogert, A., Bruin, G., Hartman, W., & Barneveld, A. (1995). How the horse moves: 1. Significance of graphical representations of equine forelimb kinematics. *Equine Veterinary Journal, 27*(1), 31–38.

Dyce, K. M., Sack, W. O., & Wensing, C. J. G. (2002). *Textbook of Veterinary Anatomy* (3rd ed.). Philadelphia, PA: W.B. Saunders.

Essig, C., Merritt, J., Stubbs, N., & Clayton, H. (2013). Localization of the cutaneous trunci muscle reflex in horses. *American Journal of Veterinary Research, 74*(11), 1428–1432.

Findley, T., Chaudhry, H., & Dhar, S. (2015). Transmission of muscle force to fascia during exercise. *Journal of Bodywork and Movement Therapies, 19*(1), 119–123.

Garfin, S., Tipton, C., Mubarak, S., Woo, S., Hargens, A., & Akeson, W. (1981). Role of fascia in maintenance of muscle tension and pressure. *Journal of Applied Physiology, 51*(2), 317–320.

Kobluk, C. (1995). Compartment syndrome. In C. Kobluk, T. Ames, & R. Geor (Eds.), *The Horse: Diseases and Clinical Management* (Vol. 2, p. 808). Philadelphia, PA: W.B. Saunders.

MacDonald, M., Kannegieter, N., Peroni, J., & Merfy, W. (2006). Chapter 15 - The musculoskeletal system. In J. R. Snyder (Ed.), *The Equine Manual* (2nd ed., pp. 869–1058). Edinburgh: W.B. Saunders.

Nickel, R., Schummer, A., Seiferle, E., Wilkens, H., Wille, K.-H., & Frewein, J. (1986). *The Anatomy of the Domestic Mammals* (Vol. 1). Berlin: Verlag Paul Parey.

Norman, W., Williams, R., Dodman, N., & Kraus, A. (1989). Postanesthetic compartmental syndrome in a horse. *Journal of the American Veterinary Medical Association, 195*(4), 502–504.

Payne, R. C., Veenman, P., & Wilson, A. M. (2005). The role of the extrinsic thoracic limb muscles in equine locomotion. *Journal of Anatomy, 206*(2), 193–204. doi:10.1111/j.1469-7580.2005.00353.x

Sisson, S., & Grossman, J. (1938). *The Anatomy of the Domestic Animals* (3rd ed.). Philadelphia, PA: W.B. Saunders.

Stecco, A., Macchi, V., Masiero, S., Porzionato, A., Tiengo, C., Stecco, C., … De Caro, R. (2009a). Pectoral and femoral fasciae: Common aspects and regional specializations. *Surgical and Radiologic Anatomy, 31*(1), 35–42.

Stecco, A., Masiero, S., Macchi, V., Stecco, C., Porzionato, A., & De Caro, R. (2009b). The pectoral fascia: Anatomical and histological study. *Journal of Bodywork and Movement Therapies, 13*(1), 255–261.

van Iwaarden, A., Stubbs, N., & Clayton, H. (2012). Topographical anatomy of the equine m. cutaneous trunci in relation to the position of the saddle and girth. *Journal of Equine Veterinary Science, 32*(9), 519–524.

BIBLIOGRAPHY

Barker, P., Briggs, C., & Bogeski, G. (2004). Tensile transmission across the lumbar fasciae in unembalmed cadavers: Effects of tension to various muscular attachments. *Spine, 29*(2), 129–138.

Findley, T., Chaudhry, H., & Dhar, S. (2015). Transmission of muscle force to fascia during exercise. *Journal of Bodywork and Movement Therapies, 19*(1), 119–123.

Maas, H., Meijer, J. M., & Huijing, P. A. (2005). Intermuscular interactions between synergists in rat originates from both intermuscular and extramuscular myofascial force transmission. *Cells Tissues Organs, 181*(1), 38–50.

Mackey, V., Trout, D., Meagher, D., & Hornof, W. (1987). Stress fractures of the humerus, radius and tibia in horses. *Veterinary Radiology, 28*(1), 26–31.

Meijer, H. J., Baan, G. C., & Huijing, P. A. (2006). Myofascial force transmission is increasingly important at lower forces: Firing frequency related length–force characteristics of rat extensor digitorum longus. *Acta Physiologica, 186*(1), 185–195.

Myers, T. (2009). *Anatomy Trains: Myofascial Meridians for Manual and Movement Therapists* (2nd ed.). Edinburgh: Elsevier.

Preedy, D. (1998). Analysis of horse thoracic limb muscle activity (EMG) at walk and trot. Honours Dissertation, Bristol University [Cited by Payne et al. 2005].

O'Sullivan, C., & Lumsden, J. (2003). Stress fractures of the tibia and humerus in Thoroughbred racehorses. *Journal of the American Veterinary Medical Association, 222*(1), 491–498.

Stecco, C., Porzionato, A., Macchi, V., Stecco, A., Vigato, E., Parenti, A., … De Caro, R. (2008). The expansion of the pectoral girdle muscles onto the brachial fascia: Morphological aspects and spatial disposition. *Cells Tissues Organs, 188*, 320–329.

Stecco, L. (2004). *Fascial Manipulation for Musculoskeletal Pain*. Padova: Piccin.

Vleeming, A., Pool-Goudzwaard, A., Stoeckart, R., van Wingerden, J.-P., & Snijders, C. (1995). The posterior layer of the thoracolumbar fascia: Its function in load transfer from spine to legs. *Spine, 20*(7), 753–758.

CHAPTER 6

FASCIAL LINES EXTENDING INTO THE HOOF

INTRODUCTION

With evolution, weight reduction in the equine distal limb has resulted in elimination of all but a single digit to support the forelimb. Thus, the anatomy of the hoof and the connectivity between the hoof structures and the rest of the forelimb is particularly important, as it dictates load distribution patterns that are necessary to prevent failure of the distal forelimb structures when supported over such a small area.

During locomotion, the maximal load applied to the hoof can easily exceed the weight of the horse while accelerations of the front hoof exceeding 1000 ms^{-2} (100G) have been regularly measured during normal locomotion. As such, the hoof is particularly adapted to absorbing and distributing forces and strains. Understanding how the hoof distributes loads is a necessary component to achieve overall balance, good posture and optimal movement in the horse and, for this reason, there have been numerous studies that have investigated hoof structures and their role in load management.

In investigating the structures of the hoof, it has been demonstrated how the horn wall of the hoof has visco-elastic properties that allows for a certain degree of deformation during hoof impact. However, this finding alone is not sufficient to explain how the hoof absorbs and distributes forces at ground impact. Hoof wall deformation (strain) changes with a relatively consistent pattern throughout the stance (loading) phase of the stride but varies considerably in degree and distribution around the hoof with differences in gait, hoof shape, during turning and even with rider position. The reduction in the forelimb proximal hoof circumference with increasing fitness and its return to previous levels with a reduction in fitness suggests that the tensile forces from the fascia and associated skin is having a significant effect on the hoof shape in the region where they are so intimately associated.

Research into the fascial connectivity extending between the hoof and proximal digit is notably lacking; yet understanding the mechanical connectivity between structures has the potential to provide significant insight into load management in the distal limb. It is perhaps due to the complexity of relationships between structures that the detailed fascial anatomy of the hoof has not been included in descriptions of digital anatomy. Although we know the skeletal components and major tendinous and ligamentous insertions (e.g. deep digital flexor tendon [DDFT] inserts onto the distal phalanx), there are numerous smaller connections as described in the following section which promote mechanical integration of discrete musculotendinous units.

This chapter briefly describes the fascial connections extending between the hoof and the proximal digit. By doing so, it aims to present a clearer understanding into how the hoof manages and distributes such high loads and accelerations during locomotion.

SUPERFICIAL FASCIA

The superficial fascia of the hoof demonstrates no remarkable features. Over the dorsal aspect it exists as a continuation of the superficial fascia of the proximal digit and is intimately and strongly integrated with the coronary dermis. Over the medial and lateral aspects, it blends with the perichondrium of the hoof cartilage before integrating with the coronary dermis distal to this (**Figs. 6.1** and **6.2**).

As described in the previous chapter, the superficial fascia over the palmar aspect of the proximal digit integrates with the digital cushion (**Figs. 6.3–6.7**). In this way, the superficial fascia becomes indistinct from the deep fascial layers and ligamentous structures described in the following.

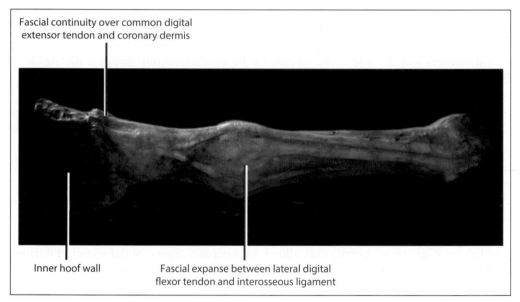

Fascial continuity over common digital extensor tendon and coronary dermis

Inner hoof wall

Fascial expanse between lateral digital flexor tendon and interosseous ligament

Fig. 6.1 **Lateral aspect of left distal forelimb with hoof wall removed.**

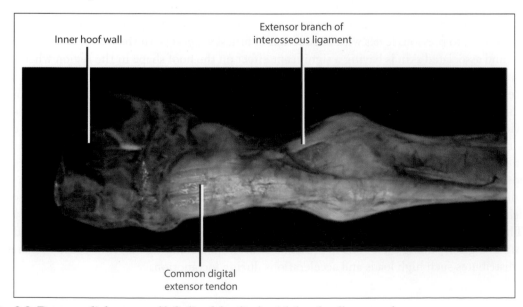

Inner hoof wall

Extensor branch of interosseous ligament

Common digital extensor tendon

Fig. 6.2 **Dorsomedial aspect of left distal forelimb with hoof wall removed.**

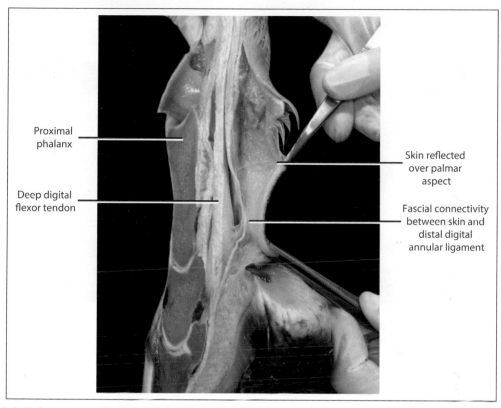

Proximal phalanx

Deep digital flexor tendon

Skin reflected over palmar aspect

Fascial connectivity between skin and distal digital annular ligament

Fig. 6.3 Palmar view of left distal forelimb cut in mid-sagittal section.

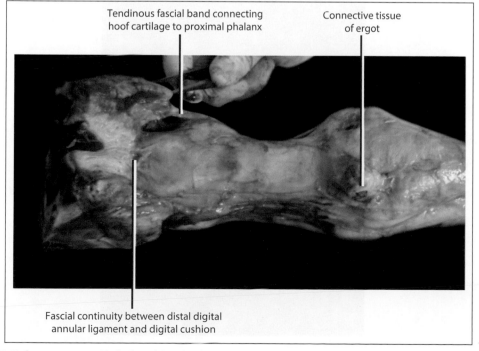

Tendinous fascial band connecting hoof cartilage to proximal phalanx

Connective tissue of ergot

Fascial continuity between distal digital annular ligament and digital cushion

Fig. 6.4 Palmar aspect of left distal forelimb with hoof wall removed.

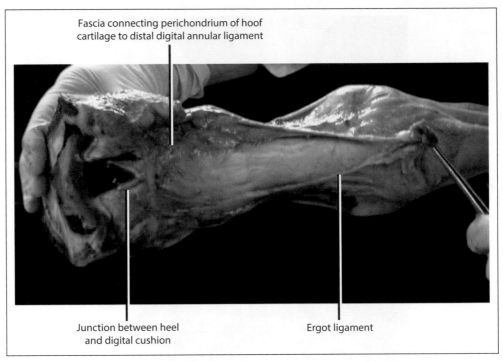

Fascia connecting perichondrium of hoof cartilage to distal digital annular ligament

Junction between heel and digital cushion

Ergot ligament

Fig. 6.5 Palmar aspect of left distal forelimb with hoof wall removed. Proximally directed pull on ergot tissue shows tension in ergot ligaments.

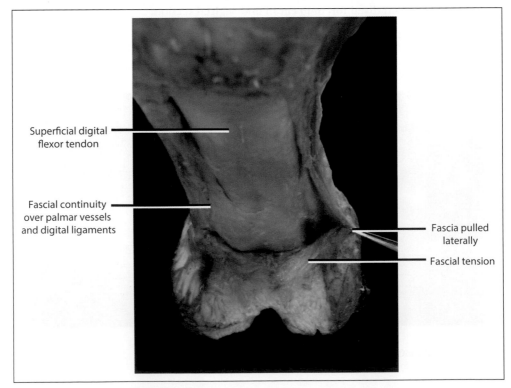

Superficial digital flexor tendon

Fascial continuity over palmar vessels and digital ligaments

Fascia pulled laterally

Fascial tension

Fig. 6.6 Palmar aspect of distal forelimb.

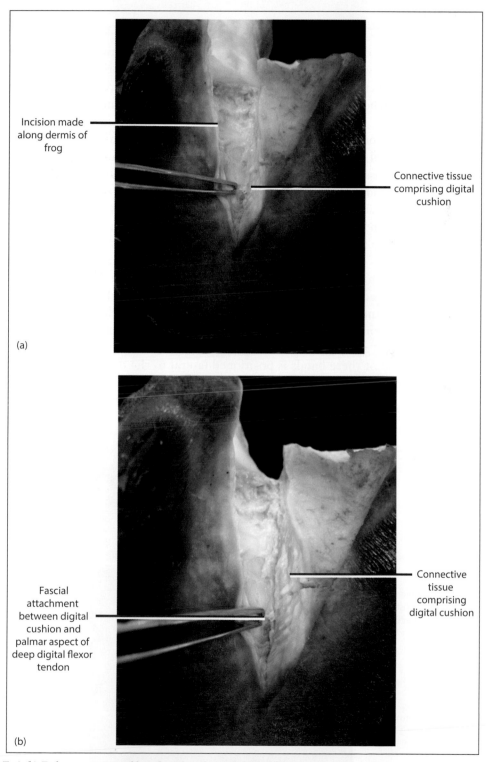

Incision made along dermis of frog

Connective tissue comprising digital cushion

(a)

Fascial attachment between digital cushion and palmar aspect of deep digital flexor tendon

Connective tissue comprising digital cushion

(b)

Fig. 6.7 (a,b) Palmar aspect of hoof with sole and frog removed.

DEEP FASCIA

In general, the deep fascia of the hoof forms an extensive mechanical network, which connects all the structures of the hoof with each other and with the structures comprising the proximal digit. Although a range of distinct ligaments of the digit have been described previously, investigation of the fascia has highlighted how these structures are very much made continuous with each other via the deep fascia.

The deep fascia was found to be most prominent on the palmar aspect of the distal digit where it formed the digital cushion. Here, it appeared to be laid down in indefinable layers which formed a compressive mass that was thickest in the region of the frog and thinned laterally and medially on either side and dorsally (**Figs. 6.8–6.10**). Superficially, the deep fascia of the digital cushion was indistinguishable from the superficial fascia and the dermis of the hoof. On its deep surface, the digital cushion was loosely connected to the distal digital annular ligament. **Figs. 6.9** and **6.10** demonstrate this relationship (as well as the variable thickness of the cushion) over the entire frog region.

After incising through the midline of the frog, the fascia of the digital cushion can be followed laterally and medially where it integrates with the perichondrium of the hoof cartilage over the palmar and deep (inner) surfaces (**Figs. 6.10** through **6.12**, **6.14**, and **6.15**). In addition to this, it forms a number of ligamentous-like fascial bands connecting the hoof cartilage, digital cushion and digital annular ligament to the middle phalanx (**Figs. 6.13** and **6.15**). The most medial of these bands is positioned lateral to the distal digital annular ligament and becomes continuous with the edge of the distal digital annular ligament at its distal

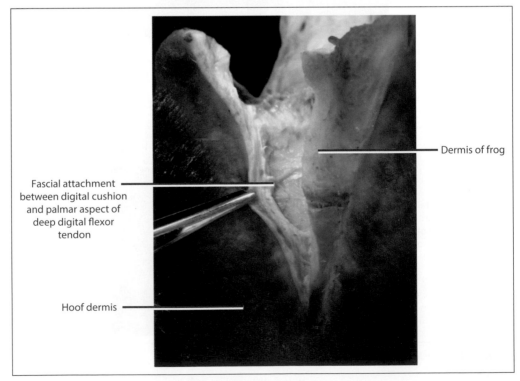

Fascial attachment
between digital cushion
and palmar aspect of
deep digital flexor
tendon

Dermis of frog

Hoof dermis

Fig. 6.8 **Palmar aspect of hoof with sole and frog removed.**

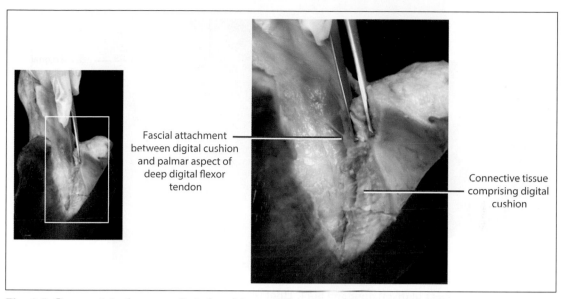

Fascial attachment between digital cushion and palmar aspect of deep digital flexor tendon

Connective tissue comprising digital cushion

Fig. 6.9 **Connectivity between digital cushion and deep digital flexor tendon. Hoof sole has been removed.**

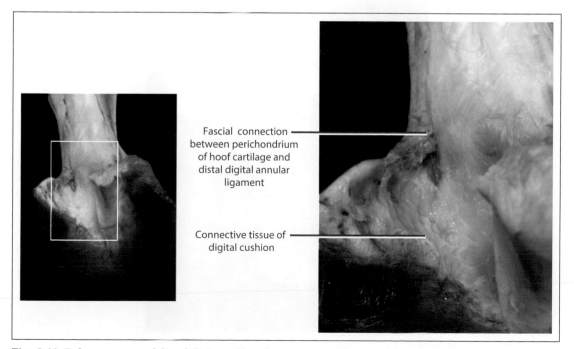

Fascial connection between perichondrium of hoof cartilage and distal digital annular ligament

Connective tissue of digital cushion

Fig. 6.10 **Palmar aspect of distal digit and hoof.**

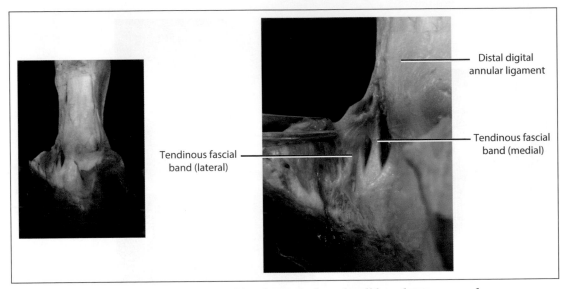

Distal digital
annular ligament

Tendinous fascial
band (medial)

Tendinous fascial
band (lateral)

Fig. 6.11 Palmar aspect of distal digit and hoof. Hoof sole and wall have been removed.

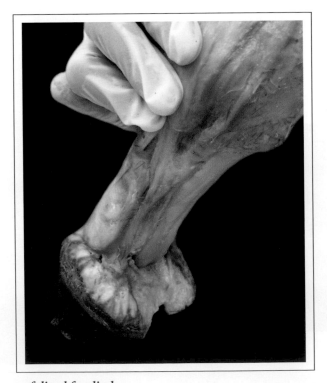

Fig. 6.12 Lateral aspect of distal forelimb.

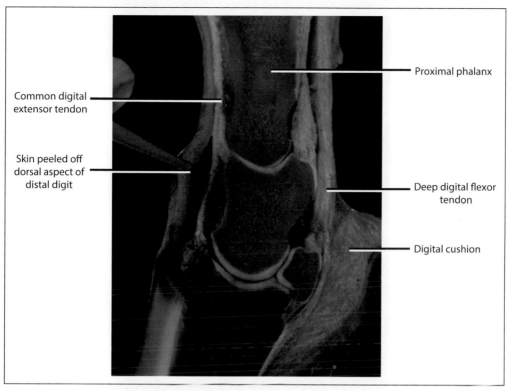

Proximal phalanx

Common digital
extensor tendon

Skin peeled off
dorsal aspect of
distal digit

Deep digital flexor
tendon

Digital cushion

Fig. 6.13 Mid-sagittal section of distal limb.

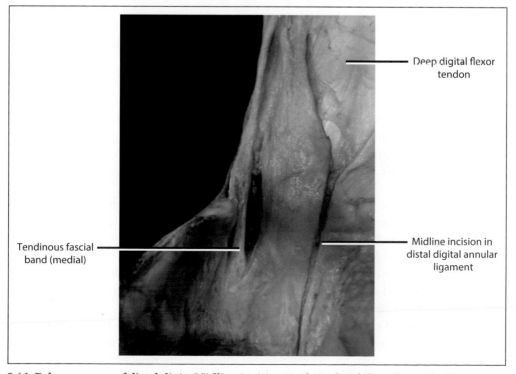

Deep digital flexor
tendon

Tendinous fascial
band (medial)

Midline incision in
distal digital annular
ligament

Fig. 6.14 Palmar aspect of distal digit. Midline incision made in distal digital annular ligament.

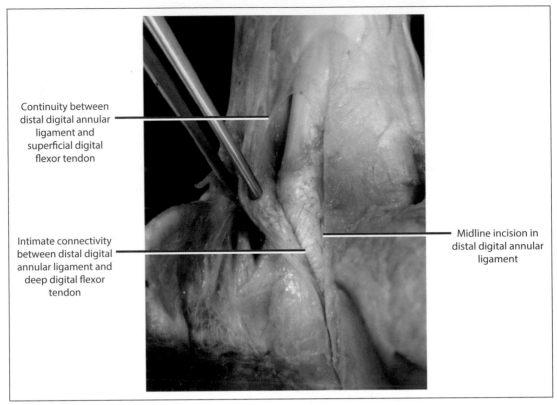

Continuity between distal digital annular ligament and superficial digital flexor tendon

Intimate connectivity between distal digital annular ligament and deep digital flexor tendon

Midline incision in distal digital annular ligament

Fig. 6.15 Palmar aspect of distal digit. Incision has been made along midline of distal digital annular ligament.

boundary (**Figs. 6.11** and **6.15**). **Fig. 6.13** further demonstrates how this band bifurcates to form a medial branch which attaches to the perichondrium of the hoof cartilage. Proximally, it continues as a reinforced fascial band and blends with the fascia and annular ligaments of the fetlock joint; whilst dorsally it joins with the distal pastern bands and the collateral ligaments of the pastern joint. The fascia extending from these bands becomes indistinguishable from the dermal layer of the hoof over the dorsal, dorsomedial and dorsolateral aspects (**Figs. 6.14** and **6.15**).

Making a longitudinal incision along the midline of the digital annular ligament reveals that the ligament becomes intimately associated with the DDFT at the approximate level of the hoof cartilage (**Figs. 6.15** and **6.16**). At that level, it was further observed that the fibres of the DDFT were variable in their direction.

A prominent fascial connection also exists between the lateral and medial edges of the DDFT, the overlying distal digital annular ligament, as well as with the fascia extending distally from the proximal digital annular ligament (**Figs. 6.16** and **6.17**).

Lastly, investigation of the fascia through a sagittal section highlights the structural connection between the palmar aspect of the middle phalanx, the lateral aspect of the first phalanx and the dorsal aspect of the proximal interphalangeal joint via the navicular suspensory ligament (**Figs. 6.18** and **6.19**).

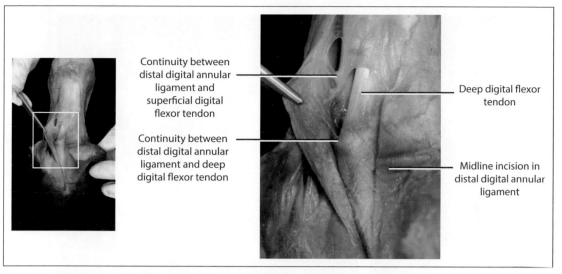

Continuity between distal digital annular ligament and superficial digital flexor tendon

Continuity between distal digital annular ligament and deep digital flexor tendon

Deep digital flexor tendon

Midline incision in distal digital annular ligament

Fig. 6.16 Palmar aspect of distal digit and hoof with hoof wall and sole removed. Incision has been made along midline of distal digital annular ligament.

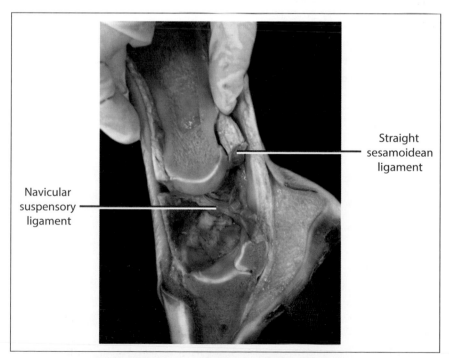

Straight sesamoidean ligament

Navicular suspensory ligament

Fig. 6.17 Mid-sagittal section of distal forelimb. Middle phalanx has been removed.

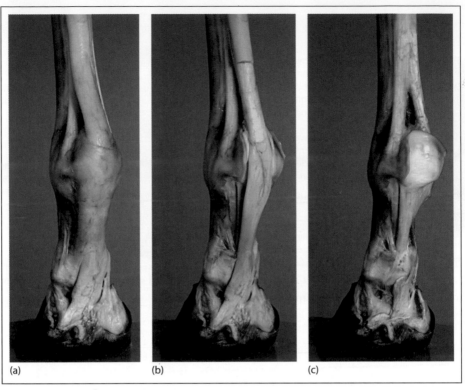

(a)   (b)   (c)

Fig. 6.18 Sequential dissections of the distal forelimb showing the integration of the flexor tendons and the sesamoidean ligaments with the structures comprising the hoof. Hoof capsule has been removed over all aspects except the base. (a) All tendons intact, (b) Superficial digital flexor tendon removed, (c) Superficial and deep digital flexor tendons removed.

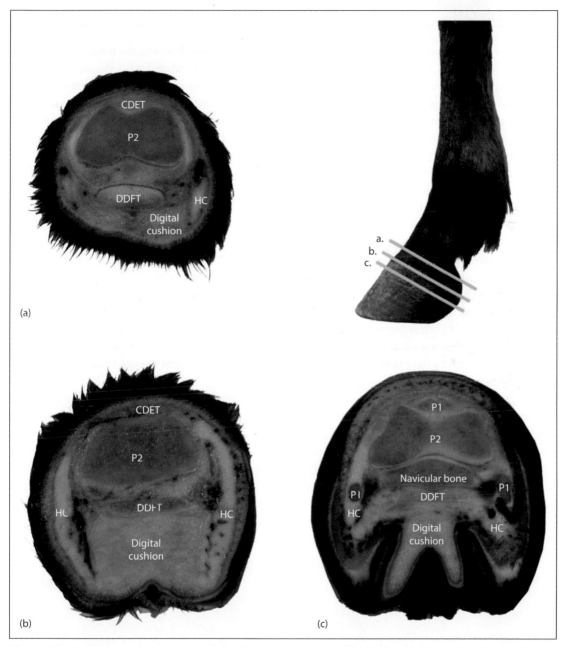

Fig. 6.19 Transverse cross section of the distal equine digit (a) proximal to the coronary band, (b) at the level of the coronary band and (c) distal to the coronary band. P1 = proximal phalanx, P2 = middle phalanx, HC = hoof cartilage, SDFT = superficial digital flexor tendon, DDFT = deep digital flexor tendon, CDET = common digital extensor tendon.

CONCLUSION

Overall the fascial layers of the digit as they extend into the hoof become even more complex in their fibre directions and interconnectedness and strongly inter-related with the dermis, digital cushion and the perichondrium of the hoof cartilages. It seems likely that this complexity has developed to mechanically dampen and redistribute any minor slips or tilts in the hoof during stance and hence ensure that the loads on the more proximal joints are as predictable as possible and minimally affected by variations in the working surface. It is also likely that such a redistribution of tension assists in maintaining blood flow and balancing fluid pressures throughout the digit; as well as promoting an even-enough compression on the first phalanx and navicular bone to ensure that they maintain their density and shape, hence minimising the risk of fracture. Fracture of the distal edge of P1 is relatively infrequent despite its apparently highly susceptible shape (**Fig. 6.20**).

The complex inter-connectedness of the fascial layers as they approach the distal interphalangeal joint and enter the hoof suggest that a change in the habitual muscle use in the proximal limb that encourages a change in the hoof loading for whatever reason will directly change the loading on these structures and hence cause changes in the fluid flow and in bone porosity.

That the loading of the distal forelimb must be intrinsically controlled by passive factors at least during impact is clear because the active neurophysiological response time (time required for a reflexive muscular response to a stimulus) has been estimated to be around 30 ms and may be a lot slower than that as the majority of nerve fibres in the palmar digital nerves are non-myelinated and hence might have a transmission rate of less than 2 ms^{-1}.

It seems that the passive mechanical distribution of tension through the fascia and related structures in the hoof is generally an effective system of managing such enormous loads and accelerations. This is supported by the fact that catastrophic breakdown of the distal limb is relatively rare and mostly occurs in the distal metacarpus and on turns towards the end of a race when the upper limb muscles might be expected to be fatigued. Such fatigue would reduce the tensional support to the metacarpus through reducing the tension in the strong lateral connections of the fascia described previously. This would then promote lateral bending of that region of the metacarpus, which might be expected to create the lateral metacarpal epicondylar fractures that are the most commonly seen fractures in Thoroughbred racehorses.

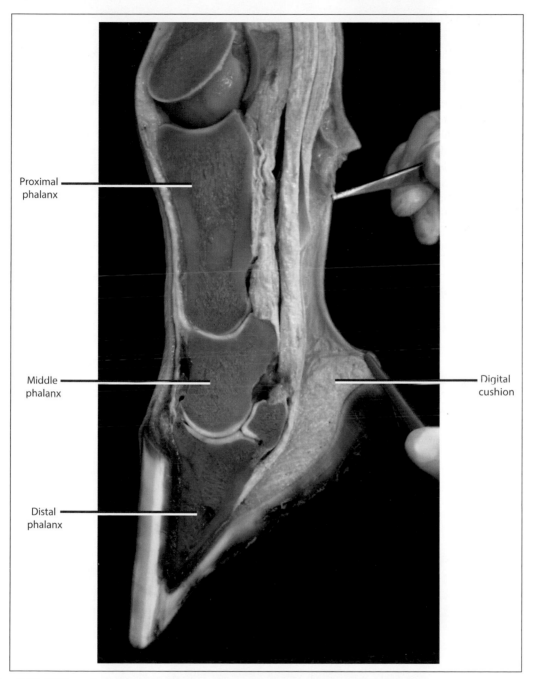

Fig. 6.20 **Mid-sagittal section of the equine digit showing shape of digital bones.**

REFERENCES

Bellanzani, M. C. R., & Davies, H. M. S. (2011). Observations on the loading pattern of the hoof wall of horses with different front limb conformation. *Brazilian Journal of Biomechanics, 12*(22), 14–21.

Bellanzani, M. C. R., Merritt, J. S., Clarke, S., & Davies, H. M. S. (2012). Investigation of hoof wall strains and hoof shape in unshod horses exercised on the treadmill at different speeds and gaits. *American Journal of Veterinary Research, 73*(11), 1735–1741.

Bowker, R. M. (2007). Chapter 5- Innervation of the equine foot: Its importance to the horse and the clinician. In A. Floyd & R. Mansmann (Eds.), *Equine Podiatry* (pp. 74–89). London: Elsevier Health Sciences.

Decurnex, V., Anderson, G. A., & Davies, H. M. S. (2009). Influence of different exercise regimes on the proximal hoof circumference in young Thoroughbred horses. *Equine Veterinary Journal, 41*(3), 233–236.

Douglas, J. E., Mittal, C., Thomason, J. J., & Jofriet, J. C. (1996). The modulus of elasticity of equine hoof wall: Implications for the mechanical function of the hoof. *Journal of Experimental Biology, 199,* 1829–1836.

Hjertén, G., & Drevemo, S. (1993). Semi-quantitative analysis of hoof strike in the horse. *Journal of Biomechanics, 17,* 997–1004.

Kasapi, M. A., & Goslione, J. M. (1997). Design complexity and fracture control in the equine hoof wall. *Journal of Experimental Biology, 200,* 1639–1659.

Summerley, H. L., Thomason, J. J., & Bignell, W. W. (1998). Effect of rider style on deformation of the front hoof wall in Warmblood horses. *Equine Veterinary Journal Supplementary, 26,* 81–85.

INTRODUCTION

In humans, common postural compensation patterns associated with the tensional lines of the upper limbs often lead to a variety of shoulder, arm and hand problems. Considering that the equivalent limb in the horse plays a much more substantial role in postural and structural support throughout locomotion, it is not surprising that breakdown of structures within the equine forelimb are some of the most common injuries that result in retirement or fatality in performance horses.

Having investigated and described the fascial anatomy of each of the forelimb segments in the previous three chapters, this chapter aims to create a comprehensive picture of how fascial anatomy in the equine forelimb can be used to better understand forelimb loading and biomechanics. Understanding the functional anatomy of the forelimb is the primary step to understanding how the forelimb manages load and how exercise-related loads can be managed to prevent overuse or repetitive and injurious strain in the limb.

A search through the relevant literature on equine forelimb loading and biomechanics reveals a multitude of studies that are mostly focused on flexor tendon stresses, joint angles or the contact surface areas and pressure distribution patterns at joints. These studies have been particularly useful for understanding the response of individual musculoskeletal elements to load. However, research investigating the role of fascia in locomotion and postural control suggests that the mechanical and physiological properties of individual musculoskeletal elements are likely to be influenced by the tensional distribution of forces through the fascial system.

This current work does not aim to present management solutions to lameness or stiff and uncoordinated movement in the forelimb of horses. Rather, it aims to discuss how stability is achieved and maintained, and how the intrinsic architecture of the fascia can demonstrate how strain is distributed throughout the forelimb. Similar investigations in humans have proven particularly useful in visualising the correct pattern of movement and identifying problematic areas when movement restrictions or pain arises. Therefore, it is hoped that this book will be of similar use in visualising and distinguishing between more-or-less optimal, and abnormal patterns of movement in the forelimbs of horses.

SUMMARY

Passive movements and tension distribution caused by flexion and extension movements in individual forelimb joints in foetal foals demonstrate consistent patterns and relationships. Overall, these connections and relationships ensure that the limb functions mechanically as a single entity despite the degree of disconnection caused by its comprising joints. Generally, in comparison to the tensional lines apparent in a ventrally extended position, those that are apparent in a more cranial or protracted position of the extended limb are more pronounced, whilst those apparent in a slightly retracted position are not obviously changed. The complete sequence of joint movements and their effects in the foal can be seen in **Video 7.2**.

Flexion/extension of the digit

Distally, extension of the digit creates tension in the flexor tendons over the entire length of the distal forelimb. This path of tension distribution continues proximally to the carpus and into the antebrachial region via diagonal fibres comprising the carpal fascia **Video 7.1 (clip 2)**. In the antebrachial region, tension is most clearly seen in the distal half of the antebrachium on the flexor aspect, and in the proximal half of the antebrachium on the cranial and craniolateral aspects. Slight extension of both the scapulohumeral and cubital joints also occurs with digital extension (**Fig. 7.1**), and is much more pronounced with the forelimb protracted.

In contrast, digital flexion creates tension in the extensor branches of the interosseous ligament as well as in the musculotendinous units of the common and lateral digital extensors. It also causes slight flexion of the cubital joint and encourages flexion of the carpus (**Fig. 7.2**). Similarly to the effects of digital extension, digital flexion creates tension over the caudolateral aspect of the proximal antebrachium and brachium.

Both flexion and extension of the digit also create slight tension in the brachiocephalicus. However, the way in which tension distributes differs according to the movement of the scapula. With digital extension, passive forces direct the scapula and scapulohumeral joint dorsally. Consequently, tension is directed dorsocranially through the region of the brachiocephalicus. With digital flexion, passive forces direct the scapulohumeral joint ventrally and hence there is more of a pulling force acting on the brachiocephalicus. In addition to this, tension is also distributed through the pectoralis transversus and descendens with simultaneous forelimb retraction and digital flexion.

Video 7.1 Fascial Characteristics (https://youtu.be/XS7FoZl1jp4)

(1) Fascial elasticity – lateral aspect of the proximal antebrachium; (2) medial aspect of carpus; (3) lateral aspect of shoulder; (4) medial aspect of elbow; (5) medial aspect of elbow (cont.); (6) medial aspect of brachium; (7) medial aspect of shoulder and brachium.

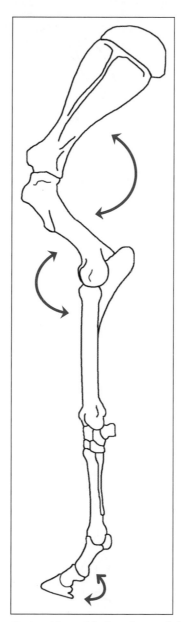

Fig. 7.1 The effects of digital extension on the cubital and scapulohumeral joints.

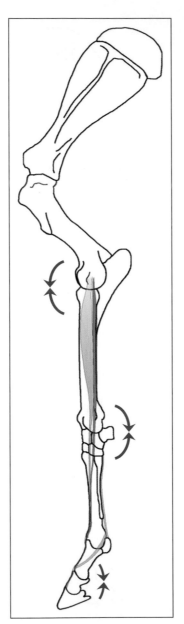

Fig. 7.2 **The effects of digital flexion on the carpal and cubital joints.**

Flexion/extension of the fetlock joint

The directional distribution of tension and the passive movements that result from flexion and extension of the digit are much more pronounced with flexion and extension of the fetlock joint. Extension of the fetlock joint locks the carpus in extension and directs tension so that the elbow and scapulohumeral joints also extend (**Fig. 7.3**). Tension is distributed along the entire flexor surface of the antebrachium and distal forelimb (i.e. in the deep digital flexor tendon and the superficial digital flexor tendon as well as the interosseous ligament and distal sesamoidian ligaments

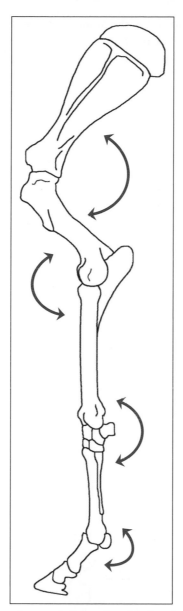

Fig. 7.3 The effects of fetlock extension on the carpal, cubital and scapulohumeral joints.

distally, and in the flexor muscles proximally, particularly the ulnaris lateralis). This tensional force continues proximally into the triceps long head and can even be slightly seen in the latissimus dorsi alongside the caudal margin of the triceps. With the forelimb protracted, there is slightly more tension visible in the brachiocephalicus, cranioventral to the shoulder joint.

Flexion of the fetlock joint, creates tension in the extensor muscles located in the antebrachial region, particularly the common digital extensor. Compared to digital flexion, carpal and elbow flexion occurs much more easily with fetlock joint flexion. Maintaining caudally-directed pressure on the cranial aspect of the carpus to keep it in a fixed extended position limits the amount of fetlock flexion possible and also limits the amount of elbow flexion that can occur (**Fig. 7.4**). It clearly demonstrates how tension can be directed dorsocranially through the brachiocephalicus and can also create a ventrally directed pull on the scapula, thereby causing slight flexion of the scapulohumeral joint (however, maintaining the carpal joint in extension largely resisted this movement). Additionally, flexion of the fetlock joint creates cranioventrally-directed tension in the latissimus dorsi. This relationship is most prominent with the forelimb protracted.

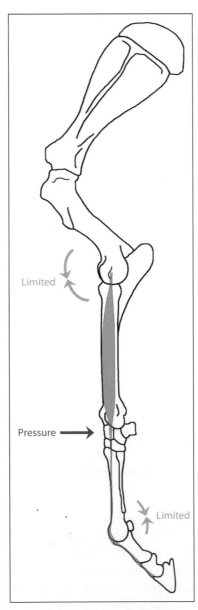

Fig. 7.4 Externally applied pressure on the dorsal aspect of the carpus limits flexion of the fetlock and cubital joints.

Flexion/extension of the carpus, elbow and shoulder

In the intact limb, flexion of the carpus cannot occur without simultaneous flexion of the elbow and scapulohumeral joints (**Fig. 7.5**). This connected movement visibly distributes tension over the cranial and craniolateral aspects of the antebrachium and throughout the lateral neck musculature (especially brachiocephalicus). In protraction, a dorsocaudally-directed tension line is also apparent over the thoracic region.

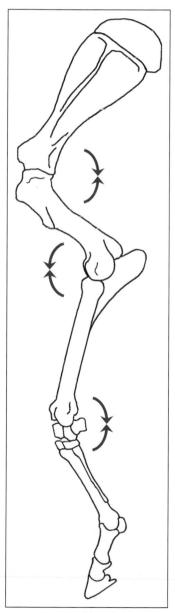

Fig. 7.5 **The effects of carpal flexion on the cubital and scapulohumeral joints.**

Notably, extension of the carpus whilst the limb is protracted is not possible with the elbow joint flexed, meaning that the elbow joint cannot be flexed without simultaneous flexion of the carpus. In relation to the shoulder, very minimal flexion is possible with the carpus maintained in an extended position when the limb is extended ventrally or retracted. In protraction, no shoulder or elbow joint flexion is possible with the carpus extended.

Fascial force transmission in adult horse limbs

Over the lateral aspect, the deep lamina of deep fascia described over the scapulohumeral joint (Chapter 5, Fascia of the Equine Shoulder Girdle and Brachium) mechanically connects the lateral shoulder musculature. In **Video 7.1 (clip 3)**, the attachment between the deep fascia and the deep surface of the brachiocephalicus has been severed; however, traction applied in the distal direction demonstrates two things. Firstly, it shows how the fascia over the scapulohumeral joint is thick with strong fibres oriented in several directions. These fibres allow tension distribution through to the subclavius and the ventral half of the supraspinatus. In addition to this, **Video 7.1 (clip 3)** demonstrates how the continuity of the deep fascia over the lateral aspect of the shoulder allows tension applied at the scapulohumeral joint to be transmitted through the infraspinatus, deltoideus and triceps muscles.

Similarly over the medial aspect, there are areas where the fascia serves to mechanically link neighbouring muscles. For example, **Video 7.1 (clips 4–5)** illustrates how tension is distributed with traction applied at a point where the tensor fascia antebrachii (TFA) strongly connects. Traction applied in the caudal direction from this point transmits tensional forces into the fascia associated with the biceps brachii. As described in Chapter 5, this fascia extends over the coracobrachialis and around the brachial vessels and nerves. It also extends distally into the antebrachium. Here, it is noted that tension passes through the lacertus fibrosus as well as the fascia over the medial aspect of the antebrachium. There is an expanse of fascia particularly important in this transmission of forces and that exists on the most distal region of the biceps brachii. Through its tight connectivity to the biceps brachii and its relative inelasticity, this fascial expanse transmits force not only between the extensor carpi radialis and biceps brachii (through the lacertus fibrosus), but also between the extensor carpi radialis (essentially the whole cranial aspect of the antebrachium) and the medial aspect of the elbow and the triceps medial head. **Video 7.1 (clip 6)** further illustrates this relationship proximally with traction applied to the fascia of the biceps in a cranioventral direction.

Lastly, **Video 7.1 (clip 7)** demonstrates a strong continuity between the muscles of the brachium and shoulder regions. At the point where the latissimus dorsi and teres major unite (at their tendinous insertions) there is a continuity of fascia which connects these muscles not only to each other, but to the underlying triceps long and medial heads, the coracobrachialis (and by extension the biceps) and even the ventral region of the subscapularis. Additionally, it is shown how this tension is distributed through the triceps medial head to the medial surface of the ulna.

UNDERSTANDING PASSIVE MOVEMENT COORDINATION

In humans, a continuous connection has been demonstrated which extends from the shoulder to the thumb (Myers, 2009). Together with the findings of the previous three chapters, the observed tensional lines in the forelimb of foals throughout this study have demonstrated a similar line of fascial continuity in the equine forelimb. In identifying the functional significance of this fascial continuity, it is necessary to consider the normal distribution of load in the forelimb (as described in the relevant literature) as well as the postural changes that indicate an altered load distribution with forelimb lameness.

In the distal forelimb, experimentally-induced forelimb lameness in horses has been shown to cause significant decreases in the degree of fetlock hyperextension and coffin joint flexion. In addition to this, it has also been shown that elbow joint flexion significantly decreases; whilst shoulder joint flexion significantly increases with forelimb lameness. These findings correspond neatly with the fascial anatomy described in the preceding chapters. Extension of the digit and the fetlock joint causes simultaneous extension of the shoulder joint suggesting that normal loads act on the joints in such a way as to provide the most mechanical stability with minimal energy expenditure. With forelimb lameness, it has been shown that the associated discomfort or pain leads to a decrease in the total force and duration of forelimb loading. Hence, with less forces applied to the limb one would expect (based on the fascial anatomy) decreased fetlock joint and digital joint extension, and a simultaneous decrease in the amount of shoulder joint extension that passively occurs as a result of these movements. Indeed, this is exactly what has been demonstrated (via kinematic analysis) in horses with experimentally-induced forelimb lameness. Hence, it can be concluded from the correlation between these studies that investigation into fascial lines and connectivity in the horse has similar potential for understanding biomechanics and locomotory pathologies as it has in humans. Additionally, it shows the role of mechanical connections in coordinating movement which may be outside (or at least very minimally dependent on) direct nervous system control.

One aspect of forelimb locomotion which appears to be almost entirely mechanically-enabled is the extension of the carpal, elbow and shoulder joints in both a ventrally extended and a protracted position with digital and fetlock joint extension. In both positions, extension of the distal joints lock the carpal, elbow and shoulder joints in an extended position, thereby providing a passively coordinated structural support column. This is generally referred to as the passive stay apparatus (Dyce, Sack, & Wensing, 2002; Ferraro, Stover, & Whitcomb, 2007; Nickel et al., 1986). When standing square in a live horse, passive support of the forelimb is enabled through ground reaction forces acting on the limb and causing fetlock hyperextension. The accessory (check) ligaments then act as tension bands for stability of the carpus, fetlock and digit, whilst several other musculotendinous structures passively extend the shoulder and elbow joints (Ferraro et al., 2007). With forelimb protraction, however, there is a lack of ground reaction forces which hyperextend the fetlock joint and maintain the carpus in a fully extended position. Instead it can be assumed that active muscle contractility and/or passive forces from the catapult action of the limb (Wilson, Watson, & Lichtwark, 2003) maintain its position. The locking of the carpus, elbow and shoulder joints in a protracted position would therefore contribute to the locomotory efficiency of the limb by providing inherent stability in preparation for impact.

This relationship between the joints cannot be easily explained by the physical restriction of the articulating bones nor can it be explained solely by tension in the accessory (check) ligaments of the flexor tendons as described earlier. Desmotomy of the deep digital flexor tendon accessory ligament has been shown to cause redistribution of load in the forelimb without severely affecting the stability and overall locomotory ability of the limb (Buchner, Savelberg, & Becker, 1996). This strongly suggests that other myofascial relationships are important in promoting the passive stay mechanism of the limb. By investigating the passive effects of myofascial connections in the forelimb, it has become apparent that locking the carpus in extension (which occurs naturally through

---

Video 7.2 Joint Movements in the Equine Forelimb (https://youtu.be/gyWiC95woLl)

(1) Joint flexion and extension (forelimb extended ventrally); (2) Digital flexion and extension; (3) Fetlock joint flexion and extension; (4) Carpal joint flexion and extension; (5) Digital flexion and extension- forelimb protracted; (6) Fetlock joint flexion and extension- forelimb protracted; (7) Carpal joint flexion and extension- forelimb protracted; (8) Digital flexion and extension – forelimb slightly retracted; (8) Fetlock joint flexion and extension – forelimb slightly retracted; (9) Shoulder and elbow joint flexion and extension; (10) Scapula range of movement.

---

fetlock hyperextension) creates tension in the musculotendinous units spanning the flexor aspect of the limb, as well as the cranial and craniolateral aspects. Tension over the cranial and craniolateral aspects is particularly important because it explains how shoulder flexion is prevented. Chapter 5, Fascia of the Equine Shoulder Girdle and Brachium, describes how fascia covering the extensor carpi radialis attaches proximally to the lateral humeral shaft. In addition to this, we know from early anatomical works that the extensor carpi radialis provides an insertion for the distal biceps brachii tendon (via the lacertus fibrosis) (Nickel et al., 1986; Sisson & Grossman, 1938) which in turn transmits tension through the biceps brachii. The origin of the biceps brachii on the tuber of the scapula (Nickel et al., 1986) allows passive resistance to shoulder flexion through tension in the biceps brachii. It is suggested here that it is also through the extensor carpi radialis that elbow joint flexion is largely restricted when the carpus is extended. Furthermore, the preceding chapters describe a particularly intricate arrangement of fascia which neatly and strongly connects muscles of the shoulder, elbow and antebrachium. Such connectivity strongly suggests that the architectural arrangement of the fascia coordinates these limb segments thereby contributing to the passive support of the limb.

Lastly, it is noted here that certain joint movements create tensional lines that extend into the thorax and neck regions. Although fascial connections were not investigated past the forelimb, particular connections were observed in the brachium and shoulder regions which suggest that further investigation into other myofascial lines in the horse, and the integration between these lines and the forelimb is worthwhile. These connections mostly occur through the latissimus dorsi, the brachiocephalicus and the pectoral muscles. Additionally, **Video 7.2** shows the range of movement of the shoulder against the thorax. Hence this degree of movement will inevitably affect (through the tensional distribution of forces) the thorax, neck, and potentially the contralateral and ipsilateral limbs, thereby having further implications for understanding the development of compensatory postural adjustments.

REFERENCES

Buchner, H., Savelberg, H., & Becker, C. (1996). Load redistribution after desmotomy of the accessory ligament of the deep digital flexor tendon in adult horses. *The Veterinary Quarterly*, *18*(S2), 70–74.

Dyce, K. M., Sack, W. O., & Wensing, C. J. G. (2002). *Textbook of Veterinary Anatomy* (3rd ed.). Philadelphia, PA: W.B. Saunders.

Ferraro, G., Stover, S., & Whitcomb, M. (2007). Suspensory ligament injuries in horses. In University of California, Centre for Equine Health, Davis (Ed.). University of California, Davis: Center for Equine Health.

Myers, T. (2009). *Anatomy Trains: Myofascial Meridians for Manual and Movement Therapists* (2nd ed.). Edinburgh: Elsevier.

Nickel, R., Schummer, A., Seiferle, E., Wilkens, H., Wille, K.-H., & Frewein, J. (1986). *The Anatomy of the Domestic Mammals* (Vol. 1). Berlin: Verlag Paul Parey.

Sisson, S., & Grossman, J. (1938). *The Anatomy of the Domestic Animals* (3rd ed.). Philadelphia, PA: W.B Saunders.

Wilson, A. M., Watson, J. C., & Lichtwark, G. A. (2003). Biomechanics: A catapult action for rapid limb protraction. *Nature, 421*(6918), 35–36.

BIBLIOGRAPHY

Back, W., Schamhardt, H., Savelberg, H., van den Bogert, A., Bruin, G., Hartman, W., & Barneveld, A. (1995). How the horse moves: 1. Significance of graphical representations of equine forelimb kinematics. *Equine Veterinary Journal, 27*(1), 31–38.

Brama, P., Tekoppele, J., Bank, R., Barneveld, A., & van Weeren, P. (2000). Functional adaptation of equine articular cartilage: The formation of regional biochemical characteristics up to age one year. *Equine Veterinary Journal, 32*(3), 217–221.

Brama, P. A. J., Karssenberg, D., Barneveld, A., & van Weeren, P. R. (2001). Contact areas and pressure distribution on the proximal articular surface of the proximal phalanx under sagittal plane loading. *Equine Veterinary Journal, 33*, 26–32.

Buchner, H., Schamhardt, H., & Barneveld, A. (1996). Limb movement adaptation in horses with experimentally induced fore- or hind limb lameness. *Equine Veterinary Journal, 28*, 63–70.

Clayton, H., Lanovaz, J., Schamhardt, H., Willemen, M., & Colborne, G. (1998). Net joint moments and powers in the equine forelimb during the stance phase of the trot. *Equine Veterinary Journal, 30*(5), 384–389.

Clayton, H., Schamhardt, H., Willemen, M., Lanovaz, J., & Colborne, G. (2000). Kinematics and ground reaction forces in horses with superficial digital flexor tendonitis. *American Journal of Veterinary Research, 61*(2), 191–196.

Full, R., & Koditschek, D. (1999). Templates and anchors: Neuromechanical hypothesis of legged locomotion on land. *Journal of Experimental Biology, 202*, 3325–3332.

Gaivão, M., Rambags, B., & Stout, T. (2014). Gastrulation and the establishment of the three germ layers in the early horse conceptus. *Theriogenology, 82*(2), 354–365.

Galisteo, A., Cano, M., Morales, J., Miró, F., Vivo, J., & Agüera, E. (1997). Kinematics in horses at the trot before and after an induced forelimb supporting lameness. *Equine Veterinary Journal, 29*(S23), 97–101. doi:10.1111/j.2042-3306.1997.tb05064.x

Jeffcott, L. B., Rossdale, P. D., Freestone, J., Frank, C. J., & Towers-Clark, P. F. (1982). An assessment of wastage in Thoroughbred racing from conception to 4 years of age fertility, horse. *Equine Veterinary Journal, 14*(3), 185–198.

Kawamata, S., Ozawa, J., Hashimoto, M., Kurose, T., & Shinohara, H. (2003). Structure of the rat subcutaneous connective tissue in relation to its sliding mechanism. *Archives of Histology and Cytology, 66*(3), 273–279.

Kubow, T., & Full, R. (1999). The role of the mechanical system in control: A hypothesis of self-stabilization in hexapedal runners. *Philosophical Transactions of the Royal Society B: Biological Sciences, 354*(1385), 854–862.

Meershoek, L. S., Schamhardt, H. C., Roepstorff, L., & Johnston, C. (2001). Forelimb tendon loading during jump landings and the influence of fence height. *Equine Veterinary Journal Supplement, 33*(S33), 6–10.

Merkens, H., & Schamhardt, H. (1988). Evaluation of equine locomotion during different degrees of experimentally induced lameness II: Distribution of ground reaction force patterns of the concurrently loaded limbs. *Equine Veterinary Journal, 20*, 107–112. doi:10.1111/j.2042-3306.1988.tb04656.x

Myers, T. (1997). The 'anatomy trains'. *Journal of Bodywork and Movement Therapies, 1*(2), 91–101.

Njaa, B. (2012). *Kirkbride's Diagnosis of Abortion and Neonatal Loss in Animals* (4th ed.). Chicester: John Wiley & Sons.

Parry, D. A. D., Craig, A. S., & Barnes, G. R. G. (1978). Tendon and ligament from the horse: An ultrastructural study of collagen fibrils and elastic fibres as a function of age. *Proceedings of the Royal Society of London, 203*, 293–303.

Peloso, J. G., Mundy, G. D., & Cohen, N. D. (1994). Prevalence of, and factors associated with, musculoskeletal racing injuries of thoroughbreds. *Journal of the American Veterinary Medical Association, 204*, 620–626.

Perkins, N. R., Reid, S. W. J., & Morris, R. S. (2004). Profiling the New Zealand Thoroughbred racing industry. 2. Conditions interfering with training and racing. *New Zealand Veterinary Journal, 53*(1), 69–76.

Pool, R. R. (1996). Pathologic manifestations of joint disease in the athletic horse. In C. W. McIlwraith & G. W. Trotter (Eds.), *Joint Disease in the Horse*. Philadelphia, PA: W.B. Saunders.

Railbert, M., & Hodgins, J. (1993). *Legged Robots Biological Neural Networks in Invertebrate Neuroethology and Robotics* (pp. 319–354). Boston, MA: Academic Press.

Schleip, R. (2015). *Fascia in Sport and Movement*. Pencaitland: Handspring Publishing Limited.

Stecco, A., Macchi, V., Masiero, S., Porzionato, A., Tiengo, C., Stecco, C., … De Caro, R. (2009). Pectoral and femoral fasciae: Common aspects and regional specializations. *Surgical and Radiologic Anatomy, 31*(1), 35–42.

Stecco, A., Masiero, S., Macchi, V., Stecco, C., Porzionato, A., & De Caro, R. (2009). The pectoral fascia: Anatomical and histological study. *Journal of Bodywork and Movement Therapies, 13*(1), 255–261.

Stecco, C. (2015). *Functional Atlas of the Human Fascial System*. Edinburgh: Elsevier.

Stecco, C., Cappellari, A., Macchi, V., Porzionato, A., Morra, A., Berizzi, A., & De Caro, R. (2014). The paratendineous tissues: An anatomical study of their role in the pathogenesis of tendinopathy. *Surgical and Radiologic Anatomy, 36*(6), 561–572. doi:10.1007/s00276-013-1244-8

Stecco, C., Porzionato, A., Macchi, V., Stecco, A., Vigato, E., Parenti, A., … De Caro, R. (2008). The expansions of the pectoral girdle muscles onto the brachial fascia: Morphological aspects and spatial disposition. *Cells Tissues Organs, 188*, 320–329.

Swanstrom, M., Zarucco, L., Stover, S., Hubbard, M., Hawkins, D., Driessen, B., & Steffey, E. (2005). Passive and active mechanical properties of the superficial and deep digital flexor muscles in the forelimbs of anesthetized Thoroughbred horses. *Journal of Biomechanics, 38*(3), 579–586.

Weishaupt, M., Wiestner, T., Hogg, H., Jordan, P., & Auer, J. (2006). Compensatory load redistribution of horses with induced weight-bearing forelimb lameness trotting on a treadmill. *The Veterinary Journal, 171*(1), 135–146. doi:10.1016/j.tvjl.2004.09.004

Note: Page numbers followed by f and t refer to figures and tables respectively.

A

Abductor pollicis longus, 10f, 11t
Accessory carpal bone, 83
Adipose tissue, antebrachial, 63, 64f
Anconeus, 9t
Annular ligaments, 17
 ergot attachment to, 28–29, 30f
 hoof connectivity with, 143, 145f, 146, 147f, 148, 148f, 149f
Antebrachiocarpal joint, 9
Antebrachium
 adipose tissue in, 63, 64f
 biomechanics of, 49–50
 compartments of, 69, 70f
 deep fascia, 50, 50f, 51f, 52f, 53f
  brachial fascia continuity with, 117, 119f, 120, 120f
  carpal retinacula and tendon sheaths, 87–91, 88f, 89f, 90f
  carpal stability and, 83
  caudal compartments, 76–77, 79–80, 82–83, 85
  continuity and functional integration of, 88–89
  cranial compartment, 65–68
  craniolateral compartment, 70–73
  lateral compartment, 73–74
 deep fascia, caudal aspect
  antebrachium, 87f
  left antebrachium, 60f, 61f, 79f
  left distal antebrachium, 79f, 82f, 83f
  left mid-antebrachium, 59f
  left proximal antebrachium, 55f, 77f
  loose connective tissue, 59f
  mid region of left antebrachium, 82f
  proximal antebrachium, 78f
  proximal to mid regions of antebrachium, 80f
  proximal to mid regions of left antebrachium, 81f
  right mid antebrachium, 85f, 86f
 deep fascia, cranial aspect
  brachium, 98f
  distal half of left antebrachium and carpus, 73f
  distal third of left antebrachium, 67f, 69f
  fascial compartments in left antebrachium, 70f
  left antebrachium, 67f
  left proximal antebrachium, 66f
 deep fascia, dorsal aspect, 50f, 51f
  antebrachium, 88f
  carpus, 72f
  proximal antebrachium, 64f
 deep fascia, lateral aspect, 50f, 51f, 52f, 53f
  brachium, 120f
  carpal flexor and extensor retinacula in left forelimb, 71f
  carpus, 72f, 89f
  distal antebrachium and carpus, 75f
  distal brachium and proximal antebrachium, 78f
  distal half of left antebrachium and carpus, 73f
  distal third of left antebrachium, 69f
  left antebrachium, 60f, 61f, 74f
  left carpus and proximal metacarpus, 90f
  left distal antebrachium and carpus, 76f
  left proximal antebrachium, 66f, 77f
  left proximal antebrachium and brachium, 63f
  mid region of left antebrachium, 82f
  proximal antebrachium, 61f, 64f, 76f, 78f
  proximal half of left antebrachium, 70f
  proximal to mid regions of left antebrachium, 81f
  proximal two thirds of left antebrachium, 68f
 deep fascia, medial aspect, 52f
  antebrachium, 87f
  brachium, 127f
  fascia of carpal flexor and extensor retinacula and, 84f
  left antebrachium, 67f, 79f
  left distal antebrachium, 79f, 80f, 83f
  left mid-antebrachium, 59f
  left proximal antebrachium, 55f, 65f
  loose connective tissue, 59f
  proximal antebrachium, 54f, 58f
  proximal to mid regions of antebrachium, 80f
  right mid antebrachium, 85f, 86f
 fibre arrangements in
  carpal retinacula and tendon sheath, 88–89
  caudal compartments, 77–79, 78f, 79f, 80f
  craniolateral compartment, 70, 70f, 71f

Antebrachium (*Continued*)
  deep fascia cranial compartment, 65–67, 65f, 66f, 67f, 69
  superficial fascia, 57–58, 58f
musculature of, 9, 10f, 49
skeletal anatomy of, 7, 8f, 49
superficial fascia, 50f, 51f
  locomotory efficiency and, 63
  skin connectivity with, 50, 52f, 53f, 62, 62f
superficial fascia, caudal aspect, 58–59, 63, 63f, 64f
  left antebrachium, 60f, 61f
  left antebrachium with pectoralis transversus removed, 56f
  left mid-antebrachium, 59f
  left proximal antebrachium, 55f, 58f
  loose connective tissue, 59f
  proximal antebrachium, 102f
superficial fascia, cranial aspect
  brachium, 98f
  fascial connectivity of left proximal antebrachium, 55f
  fascial connectivity over proximal extensor carpi radialis and pectoralis transversus, 62f
superficial fascia, dorsal aspect
  left antebrachium, 50f
  left carpus and antebrachium, 51f
  left proximal antebrachium, 64f
  proximal antebrachium, 64f
superficial fascia, lateral aspect, 58–59, 59f, 63
  distal brachium and proximal antebrachium, 62f
  left antebrachium, 50f, 60f, 61f
  left carpus and antebrachium, 51f
  left carpus and loose connective tissue, 52f
  left proximal antebrachium, 64f
  left proximal antebrachium and brachium, 63f
  proximal antebrachium, 61f, 64f, 76f
  proximal two thirds of left antebrachium, 51f
  right elbow joint, 53f
superficial fascia, medial aspect, 20, 53–58
  fascial connectivity of left proximal antebrachium, 55f
  fascial connectivity over proximal extensor carpi radialis and pectoralis transversus, 62f
  left antebrachium, 20f
  left antebrachium and proximal half of metacarpus, 52f
  left antebrachium with pectoralis transversus removed, 56f
  left antebrachium with superficial fascia severed, 60f
  left carpus, 57f
  left distal antebrachium and carpus, 57f
  left mid-antebrachium, 59f
  left proximal antebrachium, 55f, 58f
  left proximal antebrachium with tensor fasciae antebrachii severed, 56f
  loose connective tissue, 59f
  proximal antebrachium, 53f, 54f, 58f
Aponeurotic deep fascia, 2–3
Articularis humeri, 5, 8t

B

Biceps brachii, 9t
  fascia of, 123, 124f, 125f, 126, 128, 162
Bicipital bursa, 5
Bone strain, fascial architecture and, 66–67
Brachial artery, 124f, 125f, 126
Brachialis, 9t
Brachiocephalicus, 5, 6t
  fascia of, 95, 97f, 105, 106f, 108, 108f
Brachium
  biomechanics of, 93
  deep fascia
    antebrachial fascia continuity with, 117, 119f, 120, 120f
    fibre orientation in, 103–105, 104f, 105f
    passive movement and, 120
    post-anaesthetic myopathy and, 119
  deep fascia, dorsal aspect, dorsal quarter of supraspinatus and scapula spine, 96f
  deep fascia, lateral aspect
    distal brachium and proximal antebrachium, 78f
    left proximal antebrachium and brachium, 63f
  deep lamina of deep fascia, cranial aspect, deltoideus and lateral and long heads of triceps, 119f
  deep lamina of deep fascia, lateral aspect, 110–120, 111f, 112f, 113f, 114f, 115f, 117f, 119f
    antebrachium, 120f
    deltoideus and infraspinatus, 116f
    deltoideus and triceps long head, 118f
    infraspinatus and deltoideus, 116f
  deep lamina of deep fascia, medial aspect, 123–131
    antebrachium, 127f
    ascending pectorals and coracobrachialis, 125f
    biceps brachii and coracobrachialis, 124f, 125f
    coracobrachialis and triceps, 126f
    latissimus dorsi, 130f
    latissimus dorsi and triceps long head, 132f, 133f
    latissimus dorsi, teres major and underside of triceps long head, 131f
    proximal quarter of subscapularis, 123f
    subscapularis, 135f, 136f
    tensor fasciae antebrachii, 126f
    tensor fasciae antebrachii and coracobrachialis, 128f
    tensor fasciae antebrachii and triceps, 124f
    teres major and latissimus dorsi, 135f
    teres major and triceps long head, 132f
    triceps lateral head, 133f
    triceps long head, 134f
  superficial fascia
    continuity and attachment of, 94–101, 94f, 99f, 100f, 101f
    role of, 99
  superficial fascia, caudal aspect, proximal antebrachium, 102f
  superficial fascia, cranial aspect, right antebrachium, 98f
  superficial fascia, dorsal aspect, dorsal quarter of supraspinatus and scapula spine, 96f

superficial fascia, lateral aspect
  distal brachium and proximal antebrachium, 62f
  left proximal antebrachium and brachium, 63f
  left shoulder, 97f
  right brachium and shoulder, 97f
superficial lamina of deep fascia, lateral aspect,
  103–109, 103f, 104f, 105f, 106f, 107f, 109f, 110f
  left brachium, 108f
superficial lamina of deep fascia, medial aspect,
  121–123, 122f
  cutaneous trunci, 121f
  proximal quarter of subscapularis, 123f
superficial lamina of deep fascia, ventral half of
  supraspinatus and subclavius, 95f
vessels and nerves of, 124f, 125f, 126–129, 128f
Bursae, of fetlock joint, 34–35, 35f, 37, 37f, 39f

C

Carpal extensor retinacula, 70, 71f, 82, 84f, 87–91, 88f,
  89f, 90f
Carpal flexor retinacula, 70, 71f, 82, 84f, 87–91, 88f,
  89f, 90f
Carpal flexor tendon sheath, 42–44, 43f, 44f
Carpometacarpal joint, 9
Carpus
  deep fascia
    continuity and functional integration of, 88–89
    fibre orientation in, 69
  deep fascia, cranial aspect, distal half of left
    antebrachium and carpus, 73f
  deep fascia, dorsal aspect, carpus, 72f
  deep fascia, lateral aspect
    carpus, 72f, 89f
    distal antebrachium and carpus, 75f
    distal half of left antebrachium and carpus, 73f
    left carpus and proximal metacarpus, 90f
    left distal antebrachium and carpus, 76f
  digital flexion effects on, 156, 158f
  fetlock extension effects on, 158, 159f
  fetlock flexion effects on, 159–160
  flexion/extension line of tension of, 161–162, 161f
  musculature of, 9, 10f, 11t
  retinacula and tendon sheaths of, 87–91, 88f, 89f, 90f
  skeletal anatomy of, 7f, 12f
  stability of, 83
  superficial fascia
    cross-hatching in, 22
    medial aspect, 20, 20f, 55, 57f
    skin connectivity with, 52f
  superficial fascia, lateral aspect, left carpus and loose
    connective tissue, 52f
  superficial fascia, medial aspect
    left carpus, 20f, 57f
    left distal antebrachium and carpus, 57f
CDE. See Common digital extensor (CDE)
CDET. See Common digital extensor tendon (CDET)
Cells, of fascia, 1–2
Cephalic vein, 55, 57, 58f, 95, 98f

Collagen fibres, 2
  in antebrachial deep fascia
    carpal retinacula and tendon sheath, 88–89
    caudal compartments, 77–79, 78f, 79f, 80f
    cranial compartment, 65–67, 65f, 66f, 67f, 69
    craniolateral compartment, 70, 70f, 71f
  in antebrachial superficial fascia, 57–58, 58f
  in brachial deep fascia, 103–105, 104f, 105f
  in carpal deep fascia, 69
Collateral sesamoidean ligament, 13–14, 13f
Common digital extensor (CDE), 10f, 11t
  fascia of, 70–72, 71f
Common digital extensor tendon (CDET), 16, 16f
  fascia role in interosseous ligament integration with, 26
  hoof connectivity with, 151f
  sheath, 72–73, 72f, 87, 88f
Compartment syndrome, 69
Coracobrachialis, 5, 8t
  fascia of, 123, 124f, 125f, 126, 126f, 128, 128f
Coronary dermis, 140, 140f
Cruciate sesamoidean ligaments, 13–14, 13f
Cubital joint. See Elbow joint
Cutaneous trunci, fascia of, 101, 101f, 121, 121f, 130–131

D

DDFT. See Deep digital flexor tendon (DDFT)
Deep digital flexor, 10f, 11t
  antebrachial fascia of, 80, 81f, 85
Deep digital flexor tendon (DDFT), 13–15, 13f, 15f
  hoof connectivity with, 144f, 147f, 148, 149f, 150f, 151f
  loading of, 19
  sheath, 42–44, 43f, 44f
Deep fascia. See also specific anatomy
  functional significance of, 20
  load bearing role of, 23, 26
  superficial fascia compared with, 2–3
Deltoideus, 5, 8t
  fascia of
    brachiocephalicus fascia fusion with, 108, 108f
    caudal to scapula spine, 98, 99f
    deep lamina of deep fascia, 110, 114–115, 115f, 116f,
      117, 117f, 118f, 119f
    post-anaesthetic myopathy and, 119
Digit. See Proximal digit
Digital cushion, 140, 141f, 143, 143f, 144f, 145f, 146,
  147f, 153f
Distal annular ligament, 17
  hoof connectivity with, 143, 145f, 146, 147f, 148, 148f, 149f
Distal check ligament, 42–43
Distal forelimb. See also Antebrachium; Metacarpus
  injuries of, 19
  joint capsules of, 14
  ligaments of, 13–17, 13f, 15f, 16f
  loading of, 19, 23
  passive support of, 13, 13f
  proprioception in, 35
  skeletal anatomy of, 7f, 11–13, 12f
  tendons of, 13–16, 13f, 15f, 16f

Distal interphalangeal joint, 7f
Distal pastern bands, 34, 39, 40f
Distal phalanx, 12, 12f, 153f
Distal sesamoid bone, 12, 12f

E

ECO. *See* Extensor carpi obliquus (ECO)
ECR. *See* Extensor carpi radialis (ECR)
Elastic fibres, 2
Elbow joint
    deep fascia, lateral aspect, 119f
    digital extension effects on, 156, 157f
    digital flexion effects on, 156, 158f
    fetlock extension effects on, 158, 159f
    fetlock flexion effects on, 159–160, 160f
    flexion/extension line of tension of, 161–162, 161f
    ligaments of, 7, 8f
    musculature of, 9, 9t, 10f
    skeletal anatomy of, 7, 7f, 8f
    superficial fascia, skin connectivity with, 53f
Epimysial deep fascia, 2–3
Ergot, 28–29, 30f, 31f, 42, 142f
    Ruffini endings in, 31, 32f
Extension
    of carpus, elbow and shoulder, 161–162, 161f
    of fetlock joint, 158–160, 159f, 160f
    of proximal digit, 156, 157f, 158f
Extensor carpi obliquus (ECO), 10f, 11t
    fascia of, 73, 73f
    tendon sheath, 68, 87, 88f
Extensor carpi radialis (ECR), 10f, 11t
    tendon sheath, 68, 87, 88f
Extensor carpi ulnaris, 10f, 11t
Extensor tendons, of distal forelimb, 16, 16f
Extracellular matrix, of fascia, 2

F

Fascia
    bone strain and, 66–67
    clinical importance of, 1
    composition and structure of, 1–2
    continuity and functional integration of, 88–89
    deep. *See* Deep fascia
    extracellular matrix of, 2
    fibres of. *See* Fibres
    force transmission by, 162–164
        muscular contractions and, 112–113
        passive movement and, 120
    identification of, 2–3
    layers of
        functional significance of, 20
        load bearing role of, 23, 26
    lines of tension in, 155
        flexion/extension of carpus, elbow and shoulder, 161–162, 161f
        flexion/extension of digit, 156, 157f, 158f
        flexion/extension of fetlock joint, 158–160, 159f, 160f

past investigations of equine, 3
proprioceptive nerve endings in, 35
Ruffini endings in, 31, 32f
superficial. *See* Superficial fascia
vessel and nerve protection by, 27
FCR. *See* Flexor carpi radialis (FCR)
FCU. *See* Flexor carpi ulnaris (FCU)
Fetlock joint
    deep fascia, bursae formed by, 34–35, 35f, 37, 37f, 39f
    deep fascia, dorsal aspect, 32–35, 33f
        connectivity of fetlock joint, 36f
        fetlock joint, 35f, 37f, 38f, 39f
        fetlock joint viewed proximally, 38f
        metacarpus and fetlock joint, 34f
    deep fascia, lateral aspect, 32–35
        fetlock joint, 36f, 39f
    deep fascia, medial aspect, 32–35, 33f, 36f
        fetlock joint, 35f, 37f
        fetlock joint viewed proximally, 38f
        metacarpus and fetlock joint, 34f
    deep fascia, palmar aspect, 42
        proximodistal view of fetlock joint, 43f, 45f
    flexion/extension line of tension of, 158–160, 159f, 160f
    passive support of, 13, 13f
    proprioception in, 35
    skeletal anatomy of, 7f, 12–13
    superficial fascia, 20–21, 24
        vessel and nerve protection by, 27
    superficial fascia, dorsal aspect, left fetlock joint, 26f
    superficial fascia, medial aspect, left fetlock joint, 26f
    superficial fascia, palmar aspect, 28–29, 31f
        fetlock joint, 30f
        fetlock joint and digit, 29f
Fibres, 2. *See also* Collagen fibres
Fibroblasts, 1–2
Flexion
    of carpus, elbow and shoulder, 161–162, 161f
    of fetlock joint, 158–160, 159f, 160f
    of proximal digit, 156, 157f, 158f
Flexor carpi radialis (FCR), 10f, 11t
    fascia of, 85, 85f, 86f, 87f
    tendon sheath, 89, 90f
Flexor carpi ulnaris (FCU), 10f, 11t
    fascia of, 85, 85f, 86f, 87f, 91
Flexor tendons, of distal forelimb, 13–16, 13f, 15f
Force transmission, fascial, 162–164
    muscular contractions and, 112–113
    passive movement and, 120
Forelimb
    deep fascia, cranial aspect, left forelimb, 119f
    deep fascia, lateral aspect
        antebrachium, 120f
        deltoideus and infraspinatus, 116f
        deltoideus and triceps long head, 118f
        distal forelimb, 146f
        elbow joint, 119f
        infraspinatus and deltoideus, 116f

deep fascia, medial aspect
 ascending pectorals and coracobrachialis, 125f
 biceps brachii and coracobrachialis, 124f, 125f
 coracobrachialis and triceps, 126f
 cutaneous trunci, 121f
 latissimus dorsi, 130f
 latissimus dorsi and triceps long head, 132f, 133f
 latissimus dorsi, teres major and underside of
  triceps long head, 131f
 proximal quarter of subscapularis, 123f
 subscapularis, 135f, 136f
 tensor fasciae antebrachii and coracobrachialis, 128f
 tensor fasciae antebrachii and triceps, 124f
 teres major and latissimus dorsi, 135f
 teres major and triceps long head, 132f
 triceps lateral head, 133f
 triceps long head, 134f
distal. See Distal forelimb
fascial continuity in, 88–89
fascial force transmission in, 162
 muscular contractions and, 112–113
 passive movement and, 120
fascial lines of tension in, 155
 flexion/extension of carpus, elbow and shoulder,
  161–162, 161f
 flexion/extension of digit, 156, 157f, 158f
 flexion/extension of fetlock joint, 158–160,
  159f, 160f
lameness effects in, 163–164
loading and biomechanics of, 155
passive movement coordination in, 162–164
proximal. See Proximal forelimb
superficial fascia, dorsal aspect, left distal
 forelimb, 140f
superficial fascia, lateral aspect, left distal
 forelimb, 140f
superficial fascia, medial aspect, left distal
 forelimb, 140f
superficial fascia, palmar aspect
 distal forelimb, 142f
 left distal forelimb, 141f, 142f
Fourth metacarpal bone (Mc4), 11–12, 12f
Frog, 143f, 144

G

Glenohumeral joint
 flexion/extension line of tension of, 161–162, 161f
 ligaments of, 5, 114
 musculature of, 5, 8t
 skeletal anatomy of, 5, 7f

H

Hoof
 deep fascia
  mechanical network formed by, 143
  mid-sagittal section of, 147f, 149f
  transverse cross section of, 151f

deep fascia, dorsal aspect, 146
deep fascia, lateral aspect, 146
 distal forelimb, 146f
deep fascia, medial aspect, 146
deep fascia, palmar aspect, 143, 146, 148
 distal digit, 147f, 148f
 distal digit and hoof, 145f, 149f
 hoof with sole and frog removed, 144f, 152f
fascial complexity of, 152–154, 153f
load management by, 139, 152–154
superficial fascia, dorsal aspect, 140
 left distal forelimb, 140f
superficial fascia, lateral aspect, 140
 left distal forelimb, 140f
superficial fascia, medial aspect, 140
 left distal forelimb, 140f
superficial fascia, palmar aspect, 140
 distal forelimb, 142f
 hoof with sole and frog removed, 143f
 left distal forelimb, 141f, 142f
Humerus, 7, 8f

I

IL. See Interosseous ligament (IL)
Infraspinatus, 5, 8t
 deep lamina of deep fascia, 110–111, 114–115, 114f,
  115f, 116f
 superficial lamina of deep fascia, 105, 106f
Interosseous ligament (IL), 13, 13f, 15–16, 15f
 fascia role in CDET integration with, 26
 loading of, 19, 22
Intersesamoidean ligament, 14

L

Lateral collateral ligament, 89, 89f, 90f
Lateral digital extensor (LDE), 10f, 11t
 fascia of, 73, 74f, 75f
Lateral digital extensor tendon (LDET), 16, 16f, 74
 fascial extension of, 88–89, 89f
 superficial and deep fascia fusion at, 21, 23, 23f
Lateral metacarpophalangeal collateral ligament, 14
Latissimus dorsi, 5, 6t
 deep lamina of deep fascia, lateral aspect, 119
 deep lamina of deep fascia, medial aspect, 129–131,
  130f, 131f, 132f, 133f, 135f
 superficial fascia, 101, 101f
 superficial lamina of deep fascia, 105
LDE. See Lateral digital extensor (LDE)
LDET. See Lateral digital extensor tendon (LDET)
Lines of tension, fascial, 155
 flexion/extension of carpus, elbow and shoulder,
  161–162, 161f
 flexion/extension of digit, 156, 157f, 158f
 flexion/extension of fetlock joint, 158–160,
  159f, 160f
Load bearing, fascia role in, 23, 26
Locomotory efficiency, antebrachial fascia role in, 63

M

Mc3. *See* Third metacarpal bone (Mc3)
Mc4. *See* Fourth metacarpal bone (Mc4)
MCPJ. *See* Metacarpophalangeal joint (MCPJ)
Medial metacarpophalangeal collateral ligament, 14
Metacarpophalangeal joint (MCPJ), 14
Metacarpus, 11–13, 12f
    deep fascia
        bursae formed by, 34–35, 35f, 37, 37f, 39f
        distal pastern bands formed by, 34, 39, 40f
    deep fascia, dorsal aspect, 32–35, 40f
        connectivity of fetlock joint, 36f
        fetlock joint, 35f, 37f, 38f, 39f
        fetlock joint viewed proximally, 38f
        metacarpus, 33f
        metacarpus and fetlock joint, 34f
    deep fascia, lateral aspect, 32–35, 40f
        fetlock joint, 36f, 39f
        left carpus and proximal metacarpus, 90f
        right proximal metacarpus, 41f
    deep fascia, medial aspect, 32–35
        connectivity of fetlock joint, 36f
        fetlock joint, 35f, 37f
        fetlock joint viewed proximally, 38f
        metacarpus, 33f
        metacarpus and fetlock joint, 34f
    deep fascia, palmar aspect, 41–45, 46f
        distal metacarpus, 44f
        metacarpus with flexor tendons removed, 42f
        proximodistal view of fetlock joint, 43f, 45f
        right proximal metacarpus, 41f
    loading forces and injury of, 19–20
    superficial fascia, 20–21, 20f
        cross-hatching in, 22
        load bearing role of, 23, 26
        vessel and nerve protection by, 27
    superficial fascia, dorsal aspect, 21, 21f, 22f, 23–24, 23f
        left fetlock joint, 26f
    superficial fascia, lateral aspect, 21, 22f, 23–24, 23f
        left metacarpus and metacarpophalangeal joint, 25f
        proximal digit, 27f
    superficial fascia, medial aspect, 21, 23–24
        left antebrachium and proximal half of metacarpus, 52f
        left fetlock joint, 26f
        left mid-shaft metacarpus, 24f
        left proximal metacarpus, 20f
        medial ligament of ergot and skin, 31f
        proximal metacarpus, 22f, 28f
    superficial fascia, palmar aspect, 22, 28–29, 32f
        fetlock joint, 30f
        fetlock joint and digit, 29f
        left metacarpus, 25f
        left mid-shaft metacarpus, 24f
        medial ligament of ergot and skin, 31f
        proximal metacarpus, 22f, 28f
Middle carpal joint, 9
Middle phalanx, 12, 12f, 153f

Muscular contraction, fascial force transmission and, 112–113
Musculocutaneous nerve, 128f
Myopathy, post-anaesthetic, 119

N

Nerves
    brachial, 126–129, 128f
    in ergot tissue, 31, 32f
    fascia protection of, 27
    proprioceptive, 35

O

Oblique sesamoidean ligaments, 13–14, 13f
Omobrachialis, fascia of, 94–95, 94f, 98, 99f, 100f
Omotransversarius, 6t, 100f
Omotransversus, fascia of, 105, 106f

P

Palmar annular ligament, 17
Passive movement
    fascial force transmission in, 120
    forelimb coordination of, 162–164
Passive stay apparatus, 13, 163
Pectoral girdle, musculature of, 5, 6t
Pectoralis ascendens, fascia of, 123, 125f
Pectoralis descendens, fascia of, 95, 97f
Pectoralis transversus, fascia of, 88–89
Phalanges, 12–13, 12f, 153f
Post-anaesthetic myopathy, 119
Proprioception, in distal forelimb, 35
Proximal digit
    bones of, 152, 153f
    deep fascia, dorsal aspect, 34, 39
        connectivity of fetlock joint, 36f
        equine proximal digit, 40f
        fetlock joint, 35f, 37f, 38f, 39f
        fetlock joint viewed proximally, 38f
        metacarpus and fetlock joint, 34f
    deep fascia, lateral aspect, 34, 39
        equine proximal digit, 40f, 41f
        fetlock joint, 36f, 39f
        lateral digital extensor tendon, 23f
    deep fascia, medial aspect, 34, 39
        connectivity of fetlock joint, 36f
        fetlock joint, 35f, 37f
        fetlock joint viewed proximally, 38f
        metacarpus and fetlock joint, 34f
    deep fascia, palmar aspect, 41–45, 46f
        distal digit, 147f, 148f
        distal digit and hoof, 145f, 149f
        proximal digit, 44f
        proximodistal view of fetlock joint, 43f, 45f
    flexion/extension line of tension of, 156, 157f, 158f
    hoof fascial connectivity with. *See* Hoof

loading forces and injury of, 19–20
superficial fascia, 20–21, 20f
  cross-hatching in, 22
  load bearing role of, 23, 26
  vessel and nerve protection by, 27
superficial fascia, dorsal aspect, 21, 23–24, 23f, 26f
  digit, 22f
  left digit, 21f
superficial fascia, lateral aspect, 21, 23–24, 25f
  digit, 22f
  lateral digital extensor tendon, 23f
  proximal digit, 27f
superficial fascia, medial aspect, 20f, 21, 22f, 23–24, 24f, 26f, 28f
  medial ligament of ergot and skin, 31f
superficial fascia, palmar aspect, 22, 22f, 24f, 25f, 28–29, 28f, 32f
  fetlock joint, 30f
  fetlock joint and digit, 29f
  medial ligament of ergot and skin, 31f
Proximal digital annular ligament, 17
Proximal forelimb. See also Brachium; Shoulder girdle
  injuries of, 93
  musculature of, 5–9, 6t, 8t, 9t, 10f, 11t
  skeletal anatomy of, 5–9, 7f, 8f
Proximal interphalangeal joint, 7f
Proximal phalanx, 12–13, 12f, 153f
Proximal sesamoids bones (PSBs), 12–13, 12f

R

Radius, 7, 8f
Rhomboideus, 5, 6t
Ruffini endings, 31, 32f

S

Scapulohumeral joint
  digital extension effects on, 156, 157f
  fascia covering, 103, 103f, 105, 106f, 112–114, 115f, 162
  fetlock extension effects on, 158, 159f
  fetlock flexion effects on, 160
  flexion/extension line of tension of, 161–162, 161f
SDFT. See Superficial digital flexor tendon (SDFT)
Second metacarpal bone, 11–12
Serratus ventralis, 5, 6t
  fascia of, 122–123, 123f
Sesamoidean ligaments, 13–14, 13f
Sesamoids, 12–13, 12f
Short sesamoidean ligaments, 13–14, 13f
Shoulder girdle
  biomechanics of, 93
  deep fascia, 103
    passive movement and, 120
    post-anaesthetic myopathy and, 119
  deep fascia, caudal aspect, deltoideus, 99f
  deep fascia, dorsal aspect, dorsal quarter of supraspinatus and scapula spine, 96f

deep lamina of deep fascia, caudal aspect, insertion of infraspinatus, 114f
deep lamina of deep fascia, cranial aspect
  deltoideus and lateral and long heads of triceps, 119f
  left shoulder, 136f
  subclavius and dorsal half of supraspinatus, 111f
deep lamina of deep fascia, lateral aspect, 110–120, 111f, 117f, 120f
  deltoideus and infraspinatus, 116f
  deltoideus and triceps long head, 118f
  distal half of supraspinatus, 113f
  dorsal half of supraspinatus, 112f
  elbow joint, 119f
  infraspinatus and deltoideus, 116f
  insertion of infraspinatus, 114f
  left scapulohumeral joint, 103f, 115f
deep lamina of deep fascia, medial aspect, 123–131, 124f, 125f, 126f, 127f, 128f, 130f, 131f, 132f, 133f, 134f, 135f
  left shoulder, 136f
  subclavius and dorsal half of supraspinatus, 111f
joints of. See Glenohumeral joint; Scapulohumeral joint
superficial fascia
  continuity and attachment of, 94–101, 94f, 95f, 96f, 102f
  role of, 99
superficial fascia, caudal aspect
  cutaneous omobrachialis, 99f
  triceps long head, 101f
superficial fascia, cranial aspect
  left shoulder, 100f
  right antebrachium, 98f
superficial fascia, dorsal aspect, dorsal quarter of supraspinatus and scapula spine, 96f
superficial fascia, lateral aspect
  left shoulder, 97f
  right brachium and shoulder, 97f
superficial lamina of deep fascia, caudal aspect
  scapula spine, 105f
  triceps long head, 101f
superficial lamina of deep fascia, cranial aspect, omotransversus, 100f
superficial lamina of deep fascia, lateral aspect, 103–109, 105f, 109f
  deltoideus muscle, 108f
  left brachium, 108f
  left scapulohumeral joint, 103f
  left shoulder, 107f
  scapula spine, 104f
  scapulohumeral joint, 106f
  subclavius, 104f
  trapezius thoracis, 107f
  triceps lateral head, 110f
superficial lamina of deep fascia, medial aspect, 121–123, 121f, 123f
  subscapularis and teres major, 122f

Shoulder girdle (*Continued*)
  superficial lamina of deep fascia, ventral half of
    supraspinatus and subclavius, 95f
  vessels and nerves of, 124f, 125f, 126–129, 128f
Sternomandibularis, 6t
Straight sesamoidean ligament, 13–14, 13f
Subclavius, fascia of, 95f, 96f, 104f, 105, 110–111, 111f
Subscapularis, 5, 8t
  fascia of, 122, 122f, 123f, 129, 135f, 136f
Superficial digital flexor, 10f, 11t
  fascia of, 82, 82f, 85, 86f, 87f
Superficial digital flexor tendon (SDFT), 13–15, 13f, 15f
  hoof connectivity with, 150f, 151f
  length changes of, 19, 24
  sheath, 42–44, 43f, 44f
Superficial fascia. *See also specific anatomy*
  deep fascia compared with, 2–3
  functional significance of, 20
  load bearing role of, 23, 26
Supraspinatus, 5, 8t
  deep lamina of deep fascia, lateral aspect, 110–111,
    111f, 112f, 113f, 114, 115f
  deep lamina of deep fascia, medial aspect, 136f
  superficial fascia of, 95, 95f, 96f
  superficial lamina of deep fascia, 105
Suspensory apparatus, 13, 13f

T

Tension lines. *See* Lines of tension, fascial
Tensor fascia antebrachii (TFA), 9t
  deep lamina of deep fascia, 123, 124f, 125f, 126, 126f,
    127f, 128, 128f, 130
  fascial connectivity of, 53f, 54, 54f, 55f, 56f
Teres major, 5, 8t

deep lamina of deep fascia, lateral aspect, 119f
deep lamina of deep fascia, medial aspect, 129–130,
  130f, 131f, 132f, 135f, 136f
superficial lamina of deep fascia, medial aspect, 122, 122f
Teres minor, 5, 8t, 110, 117
TFA. *See* Tensor fascia antebrachii (TFA)
Third metacarpal bone (Mc3), 11–13, 12f. *See also*
  Metacarpus
Trapezius, 5, 6t
  fascia of, 95, 96f, 97f, 105, 106f, 107f
Triceps, 9t
  fascia of
    deep lamina of deep fascia, lateral aspect, 115, 117,
      118f, 119f
    deep lamina of deep fascia, medial aspect, 123,
      124f, 126f, 129, 131f, 132f, 133f, 134f
    post-anaesthetic myopathy and, 119
    superficial fascia, 98, 100f, 101, 101f
    superficial lamina of deep fascia, lateral aspect,
      108–109, 110f

U

Ulna, 7, 8f
Ulnaris lateralis, 10f, 11t
  fascia of, 76–77, 77f, 85
  tendon, 82, 82f

V

Vessels
  brachial, 124f, 125f, 126–129
  fascia protection of, 27
Vincula tendinea, 45, 45f, 46f